MENTAL
ANT MIDDLETON
FITNESS

MENTAL

ANT MIDDLETON

FITNESS

15 RULES TO STRENGTHEN
YOUR BODY AND MIND

HarperCollins*Publishers*

HarperCollins*Publishers*
1 London Bridge Street
London SE1 9GF

www.harpercollins.co.uk

HarperCollins*Publishers*
1st Floor, Watermarque Building, Ringsend Road
Dublin 4, Ireland

First published by HarperCollins*Publishers* 2021

1 3 5 7 9 10 8 6 4 2

A catalogue record of this book is
available from the British Library

HB ISBN 978-0-00-847227-6
PB ISBN 978-0-00-847228-3

Printed and bound in the UK using 100%
renewable electricity at CPI Group (UK) Ltd

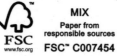

MIX
Paper from
responsible sources
FSC
www.fsc.org   FSC™ C007454

This book is produced from independently certified FSC™ paper
to ensure responsible forest management.

For more information visit: www.harpercollins.co.uk/green

I dedicate this book to two very close military friends, Carnage and Concrete Head. I've fought multiple battles side by side with them, and they both stepped up in my time of need, when most turned their backs. Fuck me, we had some fun, didn't we? But the real fun is yet to come ... Standby! Standby!

CONTENTS

CONTENTS

CHAPTER 1

BE THE ULTIMATE SOLDIER

Unite your body and mind.

AT FIRST THE village was just a beige smudge in the far distance. After a couple more minutes, as our Chinook hauled us closer, I was able to see more detail. The settlement was a huddle of dusty brick and mud surrounded by green rice fields. A brackish-looking river snaked along its southern edge. If I looked carefully, I could make out beaten-up trucks trundling around the village's perimeter and tiny figures darting through its streets. Some of the figures were pushing barrows stacked with goods, others were leading donkeys. None of them knew what was coming.

Above all of this, the sun was climbing into a vivid blue sky that was broken up here and there by ragged shreds of cloud. I shaded my eyes with my hand for a second, tried to block out the insistent scream of the helicopter's engines and thought about what had brought a group of Royal Marines to a seemingly unremarkable settlement in a remote part of Afghanistan.

For weeks our intelligence guys had been picking up rumours of strange activity. At first it was just a rumble or two, but gradually a fuller picture had emerged. We learned from village elders – who were speaking in confidence – that the inhabitants were petrified. This was enough to tell us that something shady was going on. There was talk of narcotics, a training school for the insurgents, IED facilitators. And we were told that the Taliban were storing all sorts of illicit equipment, using the village as a centre for dishing out improvised explosive device components and weapons. The whole circus in just one village.

That's what these fuckers did. Whatever claims they might have made about their desire to protect ordinary Afghans from the foreign infidels who had come to their country in the aftermath of 9/11, they were parasites. They didn't give two shits about the locals. They didn't care how much danger they exposed these ordinary people to or how much disruption they inflicted on lives that were already precarious and tough.

We did care. We genuinely believed that we had a responsibility to do everything we could to keep them safe. Otherwise, what was the point of us being here at all? We also knew that we had to stamp out the Taliban wherever they appeared. This meant we had to walk a thin line. The insurgents took up residence in these sorts of settlements precisely because they knew that we were bound by our own rules of engagement. While we had a duty to preserve life, and acted accordingly, they would use the farmers and traders and wives and kids who lived there as both a disguise and a human shield. I found that despicable.

The simplest thing for us to have done would have been to blow the place to pieces and then search through the wreckage for clues. The Americans would have blitzed up the whole fucking village, and they'd have felt justified doing that. They'd point to all the weapons and explosives that were allegedly being cached, and that would be enough for them to ruin the livelihoods of all of the other poor sods who were just trying to get on with things. There would be carnage, and anyone or anything that got in the way would be collateral damage. Bad luck for them. But that wasn't how we wanted to conduct our business. Instead, the powers that be had decided to send a detachment of Royal Marines to find out exactly what was going on. We were there to ask questions and find out what was going on. Using force would be a last resort.

The plan was that we'd be landing during the day on the outskirts of the village – where the compounds met the scrub and dust of the desert – then make our way into the village and have a dig around. We weren't going in expecting a vicious firefight, but we didn't know exactly what lay in store for us. Perhaps the Taliban had prepared a trap. Perhaps they wanted to draw us into the village's narrow, winding streets then gun us down. Perhaps one of them was waiting, his finger hovering over the button of a detonator, ready to set off one of their murderous IEDs and blow us into bloody tatters the second we walked past. It didn't pay to dwell too long on those thoughts.

And whatever the elders might have said to our intelligence officers, we couldn't be sure whether we'd get a friendly reception from the villagers. Any given individual we approached would be aware that the Taliban were probably watching our interaction with them. The wrong move could see them and their family punished. So the stakes were high, and the demands on our concentration and application immense. We had to be firm, but not aggressive; friendly, but vigilant. Even assuming that what we'd been told about insurgent activity was true, it was unlikely that we'd catch anybody red-handed – the Taliban had an incredible ability to just melt away at the slightest sign of danger. But if we did everything properly, and located what we'd been told was there, then we'd be able to seize enough of their gear to seriously disrupt their operations.

As we began our descent, we all went through the routines that had become second nature to all of us over the course of the tour: checking weapons, making sure that all the straps on our Bergens were tight; exchanging glances with the guys sitting near us to make sure they were ok. I could feel that increasingly familiar prickle of adrenaline along my spine: my body telling me that it was prepared for whatever was about to unfold. I knew that we were ready for our encounter with the villagers. The question was, were they?

* * *

A BOEING CH-47 Chinook is 30 metres long, can weigh up to 15,000 kg and has two 4,733 hp engines. It's so loud that when one approaches it can feel as if it's personally attacking your eardrums and it kicks up so much dust as it comes down to land that you could be forgiven for feeling you've been caught in a sandstorm. Which is all an elaborate way of saying that if you're an Afghan farmer, and a pair of Chinooks explode unannounced out of the sky when you've barely finished your breakfast, then it can really fucking ruin your morning.

One moment the villagers had been serenely going about their business, the next they erupted into a maelstrom of chaotic movement and panic. It was as if somebody had kicked over an ants' nest. People and animals were swarming everywhere. We were only there for the tiny percentage of the village's inhabitants who were up to no good, but they all responded as if their lives were in immediate danger. The chaos only intensified once we'd leapt out of the helicopter and started to approach the settlement's outer limits. Vehicles veered around wildly as their drivers desperately tried to escape, and occasionally they'd crash into each other. They'd whizz past you, trying to get their clapped-out bangers to jump across rivers, but instead of soaring to the other side they dribbled to a stop in the mud of the river's bank. Their occupants would then leap out and all start running in different directions. I'd never seen anything like it.

Amid that destruction derby, one thing was clear: somebody was up to *something*. And while everybody in the village almost certainly knew what was happening and who was responsible, they obviously didn't have any intention of sticking around long enough for us to ask them about it. It wasn't hard to tell that the hardened fighters had already been and gone. They'd left it to the hardened criminals operating in the village to sell all the weapons and drugs. These weren't the fanatics willing to die for the cause. They just wanted to earn a living and were sufficiently desperate that they didn't care too much about how they went about it.

Still, the villagers had been intimidated. They felt caught between the Taliban and us, who'd arrived tooled up and clanking around in 30 kg worth of kit. God knows what horror stories they'd already been told about the British armed forces – the circumstances didn't exactly lend themselves to making a friendly first impression. It can be hard to relate to a guy carrying a fully loaded assault rifle, especially when he's just jumped out of an intimidatingly large helicopter and is marching directly into the village of your birth.

We started to walk further into the settlement, following a horde of its panicked residents to the centre, where the market was located. Hundreds of people milled about the stalls, their eyes vivid with terror. There were so many of them moving so fast that I found it impossible to focus on any one individual. My ears were filled with screams, shouted instructions in Pashtun, and the constant crash and bang of what seemed like a thousand concussive collisions. Every second there was another disturbance, another demand on my attention. I'd catch an unusual movement out of the corner of my eye and whip my head round to get a better look. *Who the fuck is that?* At precisely the same time there'd be a sharp crack. *What the fuck is that?*

All the time I was making sure I remained alert for potential danger – scanning the buildings that surrounded the market. What was in them? Could I see any suspicious movement? Did any of them offer cover in case things turned nasty? When somebody moved into my field of vision I'd be asking myself: is there anything different about them? I was watching for that little glitch in the pattern telling me that something was up. The biggest threats are often the less obvious ones. You're not looking for a gun. What you need to be aware of are the far more subtle things: the way somebody holds their body or even the way they move. If one guy is calm, standing by a doorway, while everybody else is in a mad rush, then he's probably planning trouble.

My senses were completely overwhelmed. It felt as if every single neuron in my brain was firing. There was too much noise, too much chaos. The Afghans were behaving like they'd been told that the world was going to explode in the next few minutes, and I was just trying to work out what the fuck was going on.

I sucked in a few deep breaths, just to try to slow things down. Then I started another routine, just as familiar to me now as the methodical checks on my weapons I'd made in the final seconds before we touched down. I tried to break down my emotional state. What was I feeling? *Why* was I feeling that way? What had triggered it? I looked around me: children, women, elderly villagers. They were still staring at me with horror. They could see the way my assault rifle was cradled in my arms. There was a palpable sense of anxiety all around me.

Situations like this push you right to the edge. I'd been trained to respond to threats with overwhelming force. But if your mindset is one of constant red alert, of 'kill every fucker if they even *look* like they're a threat', then you're going to find it very difficult not to pull the trigger when you're surprised by a bunch of kids bursting into your field of vision.

I knew I couldn't let my physicality run away with itself. This wasn't a time for 'drills, drills, drills'. I had to think hard about what the Afghanis who surrounded me were thinking and feeling.

Suddenly I realised that my adrenaline had ebbed away. All that was left was the steady, calming sound of my own breathing. At that moment I felt a really deep connection with everyone around me. It was like I actually understood them, and because of that was responsible for them. I had this futile desire to fix all of their problems there and then.

I was disarmed: I had to respond to the environment as it actually was, not the one I'd expected. These people needed reassurance; they needed to know that I wasn't going to do anything rash. They needed to know I wasn't going to hurt them.

After a second or two, I glanced down and realised that my weapon was hanging limply by my side.

AFTER TWENTY MINUTES or so the crowds had calmed down and we could get on with what we had been sent to do. We went systematically from door to door, back to doing our drills. It was midday now and the sun was high in the sky, having long since burned off the wispy clouds we'd seen earlier. We'd become used to brutal heat in the months we'd been out here, but this was something else. On top of that, the work was punishing. Hard, physical labour, together with the mental toll from having to remain vigilant. It felt as if every part of our bodies and minds was being stretched. I could see some of the other lads were faltering and was grateful once again for the extra training I'd been doing to get myself into shape for my first run at Special Forces Selection, which I was aiming to attempt at the end of the year. My limbs were aching, and yet I still felt sharp.

We found weapons: a murderous tangle of AK-47s, RPGs and Dushkas, the Soviet-era heavy machine guns that the Taliban favoured. There were explosives and detonators. And there was shitloads of money, including wads and wads of cash in the cars that had been trying to get away. It was obvious that they'd been drug smugglers. One vehicle was in an irrigation ditch. Another had smashed into the little bridge that went over the river. How anybody got out of it I don't know.

We hauled the lot into a little outhouse, rigged it up to fuck and blew it to smithereens. That felt good. Every piece of ammo we destroyed was one less bullet that could be fired at our comrades, one less explosive to blow them up. My view even then was that we didn't go to war to kill, we were there to stop bad guys from taking life. By that measure, today had been a huge success.

We could still see the piles of enemy gear and weapons we'd exploded burning fiercely as our Chinook climbed ever higher above the village. I surrendered to a wave of relief. Finally the unrelenting tension of the last few hours slackened and I could try to process what we'd experienced. The operation had required such an unusual set of skills, demanding so much from both body and mind.

I couldn't help thinking, *Wow, this is different.*

YOUR BODY GETS you to the battlefield but it's your mind that wins the fight.

The frantic events of that day made me realise for the first time that so much of my strength came from the ways in which my mind and body were connected.

My high level of fitness meant that I had the energy I needed to stay alert. My sense of connection with my environment meant that although the rational, logical part of my brain was telling me, 'Remember that your target is in that building over there,' there was another part of me that *knew* that the guy I'd clocked out of the corner of my eye needed my attention first. The control I had over my emotions meant that I didn't just surrender to my body and let my training take over; when I needed to I could override the physical impulses that had been drilled into me so many times that they had almost become automatic, like breathing.

I was able to keep my head during those tense moments in the village square because I was in sync with myself. And when you're in sync with yourself, your actions will follow. When things go wrong in war it's often because there's too big a gap between the way people think and the way they act. The same is true of your everyday existence. It's when your mental and physical sides are out of whack that you feel lost, have that sense that you're failing to reach your potential or just end up making the same bad decision over and over again.

In the months and years that followed I've thought about this subject more and more. I believe that most people are far too quick to disconnect body and mind. We've been brought up to think that they're somehow separate. This belief is present even in the way we talk and think. We say,

'I have a body.' No, we are a body. The mind *is* the body. It just happens to be its sharpest tool.

Every aspect of our bodies and minds was designed to work in harmony with all the other parts. On the most basic level they're reliant on each other. Without my brain, my heart wouldn't carry on beating. Without my lungs, my brain wouldn't have the oxygen it needs to function.

If you're physically fit and psychologically strong, and the two elements are in sync, you're in a great place. But if one suffers it will bring the other down. The body is like a kick-starter for the brain. Its condition has a massive impact on the state of your mind. If you're obese and are struggling with your physical health, there's no way your mental health won't suffer too. That's why I look after myself. That's why I eat well, get enough sleep and make sure I take exercise.

But if you've got a body like a Greek god and haven't spent any time building your mental fitness, you'll find that that your ability to explore the outer limits of your physical potential will be severely limited. The mind is always going to be the thing that tips the scale. It's the driving force of the whole organism. If you give up mentally, I guarantee the rest of your body will follow very fucking quickly. But if your muscles give up and your mind remains strong, you'll probably find that you can tap into reserves of energy you didn't realise you had. It's having the right mentality that's going to get you through those last few miles of a marathon or that brutal shift at work.

The Special Forces understand this implicitly. They need soldiers who can combine extreme physical *and* mental strength. Almost every challenge that's thrown at you on Selection is designed to test both your body and your mind to their absolute limit – whether that's the punishing yomps of the mountain stage or the sadistic games that they employ to try to break us during the interrogations. I've found the same to be true during my adventures after leaving the SBS. I was able to make it through my ordeal on Mount Everest through a combination of physical and mental resilience. I could endure the hellish, unending discomfort of the *Bounty* journey because I had equal control over my physical and emotional reactions.

What frustrates me is that so many of us operate on auto-pilot right through our lives. We take our brain for granted, just as we take our ability to gulp air into our lungs for granted. And so we don't work on either. A lot of the time it's because people get so focused on working on life that they forget to work on themselves. One of the saddest results of this is that you end up having no idea of what you're really capable of.

What I always ask people is: do you really want to be a bag of skin and bones, barely existing? Or do you want to make a difference, not just for you, but for your loved ones and your children?

I want you to think about what you're doing with your life both physically and mentally, and I want to show you how to train both so that they work in harmony. If they're disconnected, working at odds with each other, that's when you're going to encounter friction. But with mind and body in harmony you can push yourself to your limits and beyond.

IN *Mental Fitness* I'm going to share the fifteen principles I live my life by. They're all based on my experiences. I've often learned these lessons the hard way, but every single one has been worth it.

Understanding the connection between body and mind is the first of these principles, and the one we've discussed in this opening chapter. Once you've understood this, you'll be giving yourself a solid platform to work from; but if your mind and body are out of balance then your path through life will be confused and complicated. You'll be like a little boat adrift on windy seas – blown first one way then the other – never really in control of your own course. But if you've built that foundation, you'll always have something to return to when things go wrong – which they most certainly will do – and you won't have to start from scratch after every knockback.

Over the next fourteen chapters I'll talk you through the ways in which I've learned to manage my anxiety and build my confidence to the point where I'm willing to try anything. I'll show you how to control your emotions, build resilience and smash your way through the pain barrier. I'll discuss the unbelievable power of knowing how to say No, why forming strong connections is a crucial part of any successful relationship and the importance of staying true to yourself. I'll also explain why a balanced lifestyle underpins every other element of your existence, why you can't treat having children as a part-time endeavour and why lying is a fool's game. Finally, I'll talk to you about being proud of both your body and your individuality, and demonstrate that embracing failure is a precondition of personal growth.

I'm not saying that reading this book and absorbing its message will make you the finished article. In fact, that's the last thing I'd want. These rules aren't just a toolkit, they're also the beginning of a journey to encourage you to find out who you really are. They'll help you work out what your values are, how your emotions operate. They'll show you what you're really capable of. When you do that – when you build up your mental fitness – you'll be taking your first steps along the road that takes you towards the best version of you. I'm still miles off that. I'm always going to be miles off. But I'm determined to get as close as I can. I want to learn and experience more. That's the mentality you should be looking to develop.

I'm not offering you any magic tricks, any miracle diets. Nothing here is going to change your life overnight. What I'm offering you is simple but it's also hard work. Although everything here is based on graft, this means that its effects will last. These fifteen lessons work for me. I hope that once you've read this book, you can start making them work for you too.

LESSONS

When your mind and body are in harmony you can push yourself to your limits ... and beyond. Work hard to make them operate in unison, and you'll soon see the benefits.

Your mind and body are not separate, they're all part of the same system. When you're struggling physically, it will affect you mentally. If your mind isn't strong, your body will suffer.

We are all a work in progress. None of us is perfect, none of us is the finished article. We all have so much space to grow and change. Embrace your potential, shrug off your fears and take another step towards becoming the best version of you.

CHAPTER 2

BUILD A SOLID FOUNDATION OF INNER CONFIDENCE

Anybody can be confident, you just have to be willing to work for it.

Afghanistan, 2007

Our home for the last few months had been this tiny forward operating base: a dark, dingy shithole in Sangin DC, a sector notorious for its badness. The joyful liberation of Afghanistan from the Taliban that followed 9/11 was now a distant memory. The easy sweep through the country, the crowds welcoming the American and British troops – all that was gone, replaced by a grim, relentless war of attrition. The Islamists who had melted away so quickly in the autumn of 2001 were back and the IEDs they planted with such lethal cunning were taking a heavy toll on our soldiers. Every day, it seemed, we heard more stories about lads from other units being blown to pieces. The accounts were horrendous, shocking even those Marines who'd experienced the vicious fighting in Iraq. Every patrol, every journey out of our FOB was laced with fear.

Of course, this was what we'd signed up for, but it was still fucking awful. The rations were terrible, the accommodation even worse – mud huts that had been built beside our mortar placements.

We didn't have many pleasures out here, but the fire we built each evening as the sun began to disappear behind the hills that surrounded our FOB was one. It wasn't the world's most impressive fire. We knew better than to build a massive blaze. Bright lights were basically an invitation to the worst fuckers in the area to come and have a go. But still, there was something reassuring about being near those crackling flames, watching the smoke eddy up into the darkening sky and the shadows flicker and skip off the faces of your mates.

That night, however, my thoughts were miles away from this godforsaken corner of the planet.

I'd decided I'd go for Selection as soon as I could, before I'd even put my green beret on. The Marines were brilliant, an amazing unit, but I saw them as a stepping stone. From the moment I joined them I was always on it. I never let up. I was desperate to push myself, learn everything I could so that once the opportunity to try to make it into the Special Forces came up, I was ready to grab it with both hands. The problem was that because I was a section commander there had been a reluctance to release me, so I decided to go and see the padre. He was an ordained minister, but the role he played in our regiment went way beyond just delivering a sermon every Sunday. The padre was there to offer us emotional and moral support and guidance. He didn't seem to care whether we believed or not. He did care about our well-being and happiness.

I explained the situation to him. 'I feel like I'm ready for it. It's my time. Do you think you could put a word in with the sergeant major, let him know that I'm ready to go?' I got on fine with the sergeant major, he was cool as hell, but I thought he could do with a gentle nudge from someone else.

'Yes, of course,' the padre said. As always, he was looking out for his boys.

The whole exchange had filled me with optimism. It seemed as if everything was going in the right direction. As I made my way to the compound where my hut was, squirming through a small mud hole to get there, I was full of confidence and good vibes, thinking happily about what was coming.

There were twelve Marines sitting around the fire. Although the majority weren't on duty, they were still in the uniforms we wore every minute of the day as we were constantly aware of the threat that surrounded us. I still had a pistol strapped to my side, and everybody else's weapons were laid carefully beside them – close enough to grab at a moment's notice.

A handful of the other lads were clearly getting ready – strapping on their body armour, making last checks to their weapons – before heading off for a stint on the sentry position, but they'd decided to hold off leaving, interested to see what was going on.

These moments were usually pretty relaxed. Some of us would sit on empty ammo tins, a couple of others would sprawl on a couch made from sandbags. There'd be banter, chat about home, wild speculation about what might happen next. Everything around us was so shitty. If we didn't have those brief spells of calm or fun we'd have existed in a permanent state of heightened alertness and stress – and this would eventually have eaten us up. You had to put your trust in the men guarding each of the four corners of the camp, and the heavy weapons troops sitting in a tower in its middle ready with their .50 cals to blast the fuck out of anybody reckless enough to approach. That meant that you could occasionally loosen the reins a bit – although never completely.

Every so often a mortar round or an RPG would whizz past, a reminder from the insurgents out there that they hadn't forgotten about you and were still very unhappy about your presence. Not very nice, but something you learned to live with. Our attitude was: if it hits you there's not much you can do, so why worry too much?

The lads turned to me as I approached the fire. 'Where have you been, Ant?'

'Oh, just confirming that I'm off, boys. End of December. Then I'll start Selection in January. I'm not going to be here for much longer. Enjoy my company while you can. Fucking hell, we're not going to be able to do the leaving do until I get back.' I was smiling while I said all of this, my good humour hiding how deadly serious I was. This meant so much to me – it's all I'd been thinking about for so long.

A couple of them looked surprised, even embarrassed. Dave, a tough, experienced soldier from Northern Ireland spoke up first. 'But you might be back here, Ant. You're talking like you've already passed Selection. Don't jinx it! You know that ninety-five per cent of people fail.'

I looked from face to face. It was dark now, and the flames from the fire were the only thing that lit up their features. I could tell that lads like Dave were just concerned. They knew how much of a challenge Selection was. They felt intimidated by the idea of putting in for it, so assumed that I'd feel the same way. They didn't want to see me take a fall. But a couple *wanted* me to fail. They *wanted* me to come back here, tail between my legs.

'What about the hill phase?' one of them chipped in. There was a malicious edge to his voice. He was trying to wind me up.

'Come on, guys, let's be honest. I'm going to pass Selection, aren't I?' There wasn't a shadow of doubt in my mind. That's what I believed, so why wouldn't I voice it? I knew that if I'd taken a deep breath and said, 'Oooh, yeah, might be a bit tricky,' I'd just be planting a seed of doubt. If you believe that you can do something, then keep saying that to yourself; the more you do so, the more likely it is to actually happen.

Another voice made itself heard. It was James, a guy in my patrol who I'd always thought had a chip on his shoulder.

He'd barely made it into the Marines, but tried to cover that with arrogance. Whatever the subject, whoever was talking, James *always* knew best. 'Shut up, Ant. Stop being such a silly cunt. You've spent the last few months living on shitty rations, sleeping in a mud hut. How the fuck are you going to be ready?'

James was joined by another of the doubters. 'Ant, what the fuck are you doing? It's far too early for you to join.' Instead of offering support or praise, they tried to persuade me to go through what they called 'the right process'. That's what others had done before, so why did I want to be different? Join Recce Troop, then maybe a spell in Sniper Troop, get three or four years under your belt. Only then did they think that it might be time for me to even *consider* the idea.

It was all too reminiscent of a conversation I'd had a few months earlier with a guy called Bench, the 'Troop Daddy', a so-called legend who had tried to talk me out of putting in for Selection at all. 'You need to chill your boots,' he'd told me. Of course, what I only found out a bit later was that he'd actually been keen to go on Selection himself, but when his chance came up he withdrew. Or, to put it another way, he absolutely fucking bottled it.

'No, no. NO,' I said. I could feel my blood rising, but I was determined to keep calm in the face of what was almost becoming an interrogation. 'Listen, I'm ready. I know that I'm ready.'

I couldn't allow my confidence to be shaken by idle words spoken by a handful of bored comrades. It would have been so easy to absorb their negativity. Their doubts could have wormed their way into my brain and taken up residence. Confidence can be so fragile, especially if you're the kind of person whose self-esteem is based entirely on the opinions of others.

Luckily, I knew what I was capable of. I knew that passing Selection was a big ask, so I could see why they doubted me. There were a million ways in which I could have failed, some in my hands, some totally outside my control. I could have failed in the jungle. I could have failed on the range day by failing to take my safety catch off at the right time. I didn't want to think about them in advance because I knew that I'd deal with them in the moment. I knew I was a good soldier. The thing is, knowing that what you're about to do is very hard and being confident that you're going to succeed aren't mutually exclusive. Both can be true at once.

And I also knew a lot of it was banter and that most of the boys wouldn't give our conversation another thought. People are so careless about the things they say. They just toss shit out into the air; they don't care where it lands. Once it's out of their mouths, they forget they even said it. But as soon as I was out of earshot there would be a couple, probably no more than that, who would actually come out and say it: 'I hope he fails.'

Fuck 'em all, I thought. I'll use this as fuel. I'm going to make sure that they end up talking about what I've done for years to come.

THE TWO KINDS OF CONFIDENCE

Confidence is something that so many people struggle with. It's the lack of confidence that holds them back from doing the things they want to do or becoming the person they want to be, inhibiting them in social encounters and preventing them from acquiring new skills. I know a lot of people who have convinced themselves that because they weren't *born* a confident person, they'll never *become* a confident person. They say it to themselves so often that it becomes a self-fulfilling prophecy.

I think the idea that confidence is an inherited trait, like the colour of our hair or our height, is complete bollocks. The truth is that anybody who is willing to put the work in can become confident.

The thing that confuses some people is that there's a difference between the kind of confidence that is conferred externally, and the sort of confidence that is generated internally.

When you're young, confidence is generally pretty external. It's not related to any sort of assessment of your own abilities. It's based on how other people perceive you. And their reactions will condition the way you feel about your-self. It can be very difficult to think one thing about yourself when it feels as if the whole world has a different opinion.

The popular kids at school tend to be the good-looking ones or those who are good at sports. They've been praised for being attractive or talented for as long as they remember, so they stride bravely into the world. They don't have to do anything to be confident – everyone else is doing that work for them.

Of course, later on, when they realise that it's a reputation that has almost been foisted onto them, it becomes some-thing of a trap. They didn't choose to be seen as this or that, and their standing is accompanied by an uncomfortable degree of pressure. If they want to maintain their confidence, they have to keep on winning or looking good – doing what's needed to secure the approval of other people. If they stop winning, or people stop complimenting them on how they look, their confidence takes a nosedive.

When I was a kid, my confidence was really centred on the fact that although I was the smallest in my class, I was brilliant at athletics. I was the best at high jump, best at long jump. Every sports day I'd be there smashing records. Nobody could out-jump or out-run me. But I felt enormous pressure every time to perform. My confidence in myself was bound up in my ability to win these events. There was so much expectation on my shoulders. I thought that if I lost, then nobody would respect or value me anymore. What should have been just a simple, fun thing became a bit of a psychodrama.

And then one sports day a new kid at school – who'd arrived as a totally unknown quantity – beat me in the 100 metres. I'd been so used to obliterating everybody year after year that the loss really shook me. It made me realise how fragile my confidence actually was and it knocked my faith in lots of other areas of my life. I told myself that because I wasn't any good at running anymore, I'd probably struggle at everything else too. That mood lingered for a long time afterwards.

So the next time sports day came around I was actually reluctant to even enter the sprint because I was afraid of the damage that another defeat would wreak on my confidence. *Maybe this time round I'll just stick to the field events*, I thought. I could feel fear and anxiety tugging at the corners of my brain, telling me that I wasn't good enough. As it turned out I did run that race, and this time round I won. Afterwards I thought about how close I'd come to giving in to fear. Had I listened to those negative voices in my head, a small amount of doubt and uncertainty would have taken up residence in my head. Over time it would have grown like a virus, infecting the rest of my mentality. But by not surrendering to my fear and anxiety, I exposed my insecurity and overcame it.

I can now see how much I had wrong back then. Your confidence should never rest on the approval of others. Just as importantly, you should never judge yourself in comparison to others. Whether or not the new kid was faster than me on the day made no difference to whether I was good or bad at running. His performance was irrelevant. Mine was the only one that should have mattered.

What a bit of humility teaches you is that you're never going to the best at everything. You simply can't be. Nor is it important whether or not you're better than other people. But you can be the best version of yourself within that context. Your index of progress shouldn't be: am I the best in the world at this? It should be: am I better at this than I was yesterday?

What I didn't appreciate either was that sometimes you're going to have a bad day. That doesn't make sense to you as a kid, because you've got so little experience of life. Every setback feels like it's final. If you fail at something once, you assume you'll fail at it forever, so you decide it's easier if you just don't try. You tell yourself, 'Oh, I'm just not very good at X,' and then that becomes part of how you see yourself. The thing is, you can't win every race in life – there are always going to be things you can't control – so you should avoid relying on external validation. Your fragile external confidence is like a paper house that can disappear at the slightest puff of wind. The solution is to build a core of internal self-confidence that you can fall back on when times get tough.

YOU CAN ALWAYS BOUNCE BACK

Once you realise what you can achieve, your confidence will grow exponentially. You just have to give yourself the chance to find out.

There are innumerable occasions when I get so frustrated with other people that I want to grab them by the ears, shake them and shout, 'It's there, it's already there. You just have to be willing to go there in your head.'

The problem is that a lot of people's confidence is affected by their weaknesses and insecurities, and sometimes also by events that have happened in their past. One setback, one missed step, is enough to send them into a kind of shutdown. Instead of going out there and becoming the best version of themselves, they say, 'I don't think I can do that.' They erect barriers in their minds that stop them even trying.

I experienced something like that when I was first trying to get into P Company, the Pre-Para Selection course. I went from being best recruit to failing twice because I couldn't run with all that weight on my back. Failure hurt, and it smashed my confidence for a while. I was close, really close, to giving up.

The process of building somebody's confidence by helping them see for themselves how much they're capable of is at the heart of *SAS: Who Dares Wins*. That was the thing I loved most about the programme's early days, and it still excites me now that I'm focused entirely on the Australian version of the show. Lots of its contestants will say that they've come on because they've experienced something terrible in their past – they might have lost someone important to them or been in an abusive relationship that destroyed their confidence – and they want to prove to themselves and the world at large that they're better than that terrible situation made them feel. I consider it to be our job to help them build their confidence back up.

People look at the show and they see an extreme military bootcamp. But it's created through emotional intelligence, forging an emotional connection with the recruits. That's how we build their confidence. The raw emotion that's so integral to the programme is the product of intense work *behind* the scenes. They don't acquire that new mindset instantly; it's the result of hard work. I live and breathe with the recruits. Our hut is just metres away from theirs in the same barn complex. We do that because we've understood that if you're psychologically embedded and physically involved with the recruits, you can spot where their insecurities and weaknesses lie.

Once these have been identified they can work on them, and after a while they stop being weaknesses. Eventually they might even become strengths. And all the while, their confidence will have been growing and growing and growing. It's invisible to everyone but us. And then what the viewers see, usually, is the moment when it all clicks. Suddenly, they *do* realise what they're capable of.

DISCOVER WHAT YOU'RE CAPABLE OF

There's a reason why people talk about *building* your confidence. You can't just expect to acquire confidence overnight. It's a process and takes time. A wall that's been rushed up in ten minutes won't just look shit, it'll probably fall to pieces the second somebody so much as blows on it. But if that wall has been put together carefully, brick by brick, it will be able to stand up to pretty much anything.

The first step is committing to exposing your insecurities and weaknesses over and over again. You learn and you grow until at some point what had once been vulnerability becomes a source of strength. That's the road to building confidence and self-belief. When you commit to this process, you'll build up a core of unshakeable inner confidence that you can turn to whenever you need it.

You build confidence through exposing your inner self. You need to expose every single part of your being, so that you get to the point where you know everything that it is possible to know about yourself. Expose your weaknesses, expose your insecurities, your emotions and your fears – by holding them up to the light and examining them, you'll have robbed them of much of the power and danger they once possessed. The more you expose something, the more you learn about it. The more you repeat that action, the better you get at it.

The first time you do anything is usually pretty terrifying. But that's often because the *thought* of it is more frightening than actually doing it. Once you've stood up and sung in front of those people or delivered that important presentation, you'll see that it wasn't actually as bad as you imagined it would be.

If you don't open yourself up, how are you going to learn what you're capable of?

Of course, repeating the process is the hardest part of the whole thing, but that's what provides you with consistency. You might feel burned or damaged after that first experience. It might make you unwilling to try again. But you have to persist.

What's essential is that you proceed carefully. You build confidence by taking little steps. Over time, these will add up to a big stride forward. So don't try to run before you can walk. If you go into learning a new skill expecting to perfect it immediately, you'll be disappointed. It would be much nicer if these things just happened like magic – that you could flick a switch and suddenly be much better at reading aloud. But that's not how things work. And, I've realised, the pleasure comes in progressing, in getting better step by step, even if it's hard. When you feel uncomfortable in a situation, then *good*. It means you're growing and learning. It means that the test has started. But after a few weeks you can look back and say, 'Fuck me, look how far I've come!' Slowly but surely you'll be demonstrating to yourself what you're actually capable of, and your confidence will rise in tandem.

There's not much that fazes me now.

I used to hate going on stage and speaking to thousands of people. I felt so exposed, as if all of my vulnerabilities were on show. But I got used to it. It got easier. I learned when to pause and when to keep the storytelling going. I learned – the hard way – when and when not to make jokes.

I didn't know how shit I was at reading aloud until I was asked to narrate the audio edition of *First Man In*. They told me they'd booked me in for two days. *Fine*, I thought, *I'll smash it in one. How hard can it be?* The answer, it turned out, was very fucking hard. Others might breeze it. But for me it was a nightmare. I was still there five days later. Five days of hell. For one thing, I had to sit still, which is basically my kryptonite. Sometimes I'd be too close to the mic and I'd get a shout from the control booth: 'You're popping.' Other times I'd be too far away. And I'm not a strong reader. When I'm doing it aloud I sometimes feel as if I can barely string a sentence together and if I can get to the bottom of a page without making a mistake I feel as if I've won the World Cup. I'd get tongue-tied, and there would always be words I struggled to pronounce or phrases I'd have to repeat over and over again. It was just intensely frustrating. About a thousand times a day I'd be thinking, *Fuck it, somebody else can do this.*

I hated getting in the car each morning knowing I was going to be sitting in a booth for eight hours. And yet it was that uncomfortable feeling that reminded me I was alive. I had a voice in my head saying, 'This is fucking good for you, Ant. And you're shying away from it just because it makes you a bit uncomfortable? After *everything* you've said and done, you want to quit now?'

On the first day I only managed to get through sixty pages. I came out of it feeling pretty bruised and embarrassed. It's a very public failure. There might only have been a couple of people listening, but their job was to watch and listen in microscopic detail. They were being paid to point out and fix my mistakes, and whatever else happened that day, they certainly earned their wages. The next I managed a hundred, and by the following day I was up to a hundred and twenty. It was progress, even if I was still well off the pace.

It was so horrendous an experience that I swore I'd never do it again. Until, of course, I agreed to do the next one. I wanted to get better, and I also wanted to overcome the bad memories of the first time I'd tried. It took three days, and while I was still struggling, I knew that I'd taken a big step forwards. I got into my bubble, taking each chapter as it came, each paragraph, each line.

Now I'm being asked to do readings in front of kids and other, larger audiences. I'm an ambassador for children's literacy. If you'd asked me to do that a few years ago you probably wouldn't have seen me for dust. The story I told myself was that reading aloud was something I just wasn't good at. Full stop. I'd have tossed out a blizzard of excuses and stayed away. I no longer see it like that. I'm still nervous about the prospect, but I'm definitely more confident. It's not an apocalyptic thought, just a slightly uncomfortable one.

The aim is to build confidence that's based on what you *know* you're capable of, not on anybody else's opinion. If you have that under your belt you can get knocked and rocked again and again, but you'll be able to keep on going. You've been there already, you've exposed yourself and you've learned lessons.

Imagine you struggled to pass your driving test. Although you've now got a licence, you're not that confident as a driver. You avoid ever getting behind the wheel if you can help it, and when you do have to drive somewhere you steer clear of busy roads or tight parking spots. In your head you're behaving perfectly rationally – by avoiding something you're not good at, you're protecting yourself. But with each challenge you duck, you're digging a hole that will be harder and harder to escape from. Not only have you convinced yourself that you're a terrible driver, you're also substantially limiting what you can do and where you can go.

It doesn't have to be like that! You *can* become a confident driver – you simply need the opportunity to prove it to yourself. Get into your car, or hire one. Drive around. If the idea of parallel parking brings you out in a cold sweat, then practise doing it. Keep on going until you can pull it off without a second thought. All of this sounds so simple and obvious. And yet the myths we create about ourselves are incredibly tenacious.

The best thing about internal confidence is that it's founded on stuff you can do. It doesn't depend on anybody else's opinion. Once you've proved to yourself that you can learn one thing, you'll find that you're more confident about trying lots of other things. If you've learned how to play tennis, why shouldn't you be able to learn how to play the guitar too?

Once you build that momentum you'll begin to feel a change inside you – a growth of a more general sense of confidence. When you're faced with a new challenge, you'll be less intimidated by tackling it. You'll feel more sure of your thoughts and more able to listen to your instincts, because you've shown to yourself and everybody around you that you're the sort of person who can do stuff, even when it seems hard or complicated. And you can draw on this confidence during those moments – which come to us all – when we doubt ourselves.

THE TRUTH ABOUT IMPOSTER SYNDROME

Nobody is immune to imposter syndrome. I'm certainly not. There are nights when I've been up on stage talking about mindset and I've had that nagging thought: *Why are you doing this? Are you qualified? Are you a psychologist?* Now of course I can reply that I'm drawing on experience, which in my opinion is as valuable as any academic course. I've been out there, I've exposed my fears and repeated that process. I've exposed all of my emotions, and repeated that process too. I know my emotions inside out. I know them so well that some people think I'm actually emotionless.

People think that imposter syndrome comes from inside us. I think they're wrong. It's forced on us by other people. One thing I've learned is that people don't like you to be confident. When they see it, they can't wait to smash you down. That's another reason why it's so important to develop that foundation of inner confidence.

It's imposter syndrome that gets in the way of your ambitions. It stops you from going for jobs you're qualified for or trying to get into teams you're easily good enough to play for. You get afflicted by it because there are those negative people out there who take stupid amounts of pleasure in trying to make you feel as if you don't deserve to be where you've worked so hard to get.

Your confidence can be snatched away by just one negative voice. It's horrible, but we're made so that we always focus on the worst things that somebody else says about us. They could spend ten minutes praising us to the high heavens, and yet we'll latch on to the minute criticism that they add as an afterthought. It's not the praise that we end up thinking about later that night as we try and fail to get to sleep.

As I've said before, we should all welcome positive criticism. When people show us ways in which we could improve it would be madness to ignore them, even if to begin with it might sting a bit. But there's a difference between someone who honestly wants you to be the best version of yourself, and someone who – for whatever fucked-up reasons of their own – wants to hammer away at your confidence.

The best antidote to imposter syndrome is that foundation of inner confidence. The problem is that we're far too keen to focus on the unpleasant things other people say, and we don't actually celebrate, or even particularly recognise, all the great things that we've done.

When I joined P Company my confidence rocketed. I felt honoured to have been allowed to join. But that boost to my self-esteem didn't last long. The whole Para experience – its bully culture, the massive chasm that lay between my values and theirs – knocked my confidence down a few pegs. I quit because I was the squarest of pegs in the roundest of holes.

The thought that I hadn't been good enough circled round and round my mind for months afterwards.

It took time for me to realise that I hadn't fitted in because, unlike the rest of them, I wasn't interested in playing at being soldiers. I wasn't the one with the problem, it was the rest of them. All that talk of 'X being a fucking awesome soldier'. 'Yeah? How do you know that?' Well, on exercise ...' 'Let me stop you right there – a few nights crawling around Exmoor firing blanks doesn't mean *shit*.' I did tours of Northern Ireland and Macedonia, and spent most of the time on the piss. Then, when Afghanistan and Iraq came around, all the pub soldiers left. Funny old thing, that.

For too long I'd internalised their opinions. I saw the world through their eyes. Their view of what made a good soldier had been my view of what made a good soldier. My confidence was based on their beliefs, not mine, so I was always going to end up damaged. I had to step away from that environment to clear my head and start again.

That experience meant I was in a very different headspace a few years later on that night in Afghanistan when I told the other lads in 40 Commando I was about to head off for Selection. I knew I couldn't pay attention to them – if I did I'd be importing their negative voices into my mind. I was setting off for what I knew was going to be the biggest test of my life, and if I allowed those nagging, doubting sentiments to infect me it could hinder my chances.

Instead of listening to them, I focused on what I'd achieved to get there. I thought about being awarded the Royal Marines' King's Badge, which is given to the best recruit in every training cohort. That was the moment when I really began to think, *Fucking hell, I am good enough. This is where I belong.*

I thought too about the sequence of promotions I'd been awarded since we'd arrived in Afghanistan. There was a reason that I'd been given that responsibility. I'd proved myself as leader and a soldier. You can't blag it in the armed forces. At least, not post-2001. You've got people's lives in your hands. And I was in brilliant mental and physical shape. All of this reminded me that I deserved to be going on Selection. Nothing any fucker said could persuade me otherwise.

On those days when a stray word from a workmate makes you begin to feel as if you don't perhaps deserve to be in the position you're in, think about the long sequence of events that will have led to that moment.

If you're in business, maybe you joined your company straight out of school and worked your way up, step by step, picking up new skills all the way, learning and growing. Or maybe you're there because you earned a place on their competitive graduate programme. You should be proud of all of those things; they should be the source of confidence.

VALUE YOUR OWN VOICE

There are two ways of making other people listen to you. One way is to take steroids, get really angry and then force the person whose attention you're after into a headlock. Simple, yes, but roid rage is tiring for pretty much everybody.

The second way is to speak up confidently and demonstrate to the world that you deserve their attention. That's why I don't mind people who've got a bit of mouth ... as long as they can back it up. When you act with confidence, when you show people you've got confidence, they'll treat you with more respect. That's maybe not how things *should* be, but it's certainly how things *are*.

You don't want to come across as a bully in love with the sound of their own voice. Nobody likes or respects people who speak for the sake of speaking. But if you know your field, if you've got something to contribute, you should never feel afraid of making yourself heard. When you're sure of your ground, when you know what works – that's a really powerful, persuasive place to be.

I don't mean that you should be like a machine-gun firing shots off in every direction. Listen to others before you speak. Absorb their ideas, try to understand their perspective. Assertiveness can feel like a noisy idea, conjuring up an image of people jabbering away. But it doesn't have to be like that. Being assertive isn't about bludgeoning others into silence, nor is it about counting your wins. It's about making contributions, creating a space in which you can share the sorts of ideas and viewpoints that can only come from you.

Remember that there's no such thing as a silly question. If you're sitting in a meeting and there's something nagging away at you – maybe a concept hasn't been explained very clearly – then don't be afraid to pipe up. If you don't, then I guarantee that somebody else will. When you do ask you might get a bit of shit, but it's more likely that people will be really glad that you've brought it up. The same is true when you're sitting on an idea. If you've got something on your mind and it's burning inside, voice it.

I will never ignore somebody who comes to me with an idea. Often the idea is brilliant, and it's something that can be developed without anybody else having to do much. But even if there's an element that isn't quite right, there's usually the seed of something. Good leaders should always be looking for those little gems that might need a bit of polishing, but which can be the beginning of something even more rewarding and exciting.

Even now I annoy the shit out of the other DSs on *SAS: Who Dares Wins*. Whenever we have discussions I'll say, 'Great, but what about this? What about that? Have you considered …?' I can't help myself.

As pissed off as this makes them, I think it's a process we've all come to value. You'll never have all the answers to all the questions. Some people take it personally when their ideas get criticised or modified. That's the wrong way to look at it. Confident people don't mind being challenged like this. Like the DSs, they know that the best environments are collaborative. Everybody contributes something that reflects their knowledge and experience, and the end result is all the better for it.

THE FAÇADE OF CONFIDENCE

Some people hide behind what looks like confidence. They know all the tricks you need to project it: their backs are straight, their voices loud, their handshakes firm. They talk about how great they are, how much they earn, how many sexual partners they've had. And yet all of this is a façade designed to disguise how hollow and scared they really are. They're arrogant, not truly confident. Unlike confident people, arrogant people don't really know themselves. They might *think* they're the dog's bits, but they don't *know* that. They haven't tested the limits of their psychological and physical abilities. Their arrogance is a way of hiding their fear of what they'd find if they did. And when you haven't made that effort, people can use your flaws or your imperfections against you.

You can hide behind a false façade of confidence for years. But I guarantee that one day the time will come when you can't hide anymore. That gap between who you are and who you say you are will be revealed and, like a black hole, it will destroy everything around it. So why waste time living a lie?

ETERNAL RENEWAL

Like much that's worthwhile, you should see building confidence as a lifelong project. If you rest on your laurels and stop trying new things, if you stop testing yourself, then you're creating a space for that doubt and lack of confidence to creep in. Your confidence will weaken. Don't become someone who looks back to when they were younger and then says, almost as if they're surprised, 'Oh, yes, I used to be confident.' Complacency is the enemy of that true inner confidence.

I'm willing to give anything a go because I know that it doesn't matter if I fail, or even if I make a fool of myself. I'll learn from it, move on and emerge stronger. I'm addicted to trying new things. That's why I bounce around from project to project – books, TV, business, adventures. It means I can test myself all the time. If I just stayed within one bubble I know I'd end up trapped and my confidence would begin to shrink. I don't want to get tunnel vision and convince myself

I'm only good at one thing. That inevitably means I'll fall flat on my arse from time to time. I'll realise that there are things that, no matter how I try, I'm never going to be very good at. I can live with that.

LESSONS

Your confidence should be based on what you know you're capable of, not the opinions of others. When you have internal confidence you'll be more resilient, more willing to try new things, and you'll be able to take whatever life throws at you in your stride.

Confidence is not a natural trait. Confidence isn't a quality that some people are born with and others aren't. *Everyone* who is willing to put the right work in can become confident. Don't wait for somebody else to tell you what you're capable of; go out there straight away and prove it to yourself.

You won't become confident overnight. Nothing worth anything comes together instantly. You build your confidence step by step.

No setback is ever final. The process of building your confidence slowly but surely can help us address those traumatic experiences in our past that are stopping us from enjoying our future.

Imposter syndrome is forced on us by other people's negativity. Fight back by reminding yourself of everything you've achieved and everything you're capable of.

Building your confidence isn't the work of a day, it's the work of a lifetime. If you rest on your laurels for too long, you'll find that your confidence starts to ebb away. Never stop challenging yourself. If you're feeling uncomfortable, you're heading in the right direction.

CHAPTER 3

BE AUTHENTIC

Live the way you want. Don't change the way you behave or think just to fit somebody else's agenda.

IT TOOK ME a long time to work out who I really was. Too long, if I'm going to be honest. For a while I was lost. I tried to fit in with people whose values I didn't share, and I ended up hating myself for it. I was lucky that life sent a couple of jolts my way.

I wrote in *First Man In* about the kinship I felt with the French Foreign Legion when we were stationed near them in Macedonia. When I hung out with them I could reconnect with the kid I'd been in France, the kid who'd drunk coffee in cafés, who chatted happily with strangers in the street. It was nice to just sit there and not have to pretend to be somebody I wasn't. That helped me begin to realise how unhappy I was being pressured to be the person other people wanted me to be. That was the first crack in the wall.

Another came in an incident I haven't talked about before. One afternoon, not long after we'd returned from our six months in the Balkans, I walked into the squadron bar. The first thing I saw was a staff sergeant, a man in his mid-thirties, drinking piss out of a tatty old desert boot. I stared at him in disbelief as dark yellow urine dribbled down his chin and onto his shirt. The lads he was with cheered, then jerked their pint glasses violently upwards so that their drinks flew into the air like a cluster of fizzy amber fountains. Seconds later they were all soaked, but they didn't seem to care – to them that staff sergeant was a hero. At first I felt a revulsion at what I'd just seen. Then I thought, *If I continue on this road for another fifteen years, that could be me.* This scared the hell out of me. The next day I put my notice in. I knew that I had a choice. I could either pull myself out of that round hole or stay in it forever.

I didn't change enough. There may have been cracks in the wall but it was still standing. That's how strong the desire to fit in at all costs can be. I carried on getting drunk and lairy once I'd joined the police. I cheated on my exams. I found myself drink-driving. I was living as somebody who wasn't me, but who had control of me. Meeting Emilie made a difference, as did my time in the Royal Marines and the SBS, but I emerged from the armed forces as someone who had not managed to get a hold of who they really were. I was still too easily swayed by the opinions of others. I was still too eager to please. I invariably followed the path of least resistance, even when I knew deep down that it was the wrong route for me to take.

I remember being with a few mates in a Chelmsford nightclub during my fighting days, young and dumb and all pissed-up in the VIP area. The wake-up call of being sent to prison was still a year or two in the future and we were just doing our normal thing – smashing back vodka, and becoming louder and more obnoxious with every minute that passed.

An hour or so after our group had arrived a couple of lads came in. Initially they seemed happy to drink and keep themselves to themselves. I barely even noticed their presence. After a while, though, I experienced that uncomfortable prickle you get down your spine when you *know* you're being watched. One of them must have clocked that I was in decent shape. He was staring at me, and I could see him whispering something into his mate's ear. They both laughed. Then they stood up and came over to our table.

'Arm wrestle, mate?'

And I just thought, *Fuck's sake. Here we go.* I'd been in these sorts of situations before. Nothing good ever came of them.

But it's also the kind of thing that's easier to do than not do. I didn't want to look like an arsehole by saying No, and the guy was clearly on a bit of a mission. So that was that. He didn't look much – he was quite a slim character – but I could tell that he had that wiry strength that would make him an awkward opponent. By the time we'd cleared space among the collection of empty bottles on our table, a decent-sized crowd had gathered. They pressed close to us, exuding a heady cocktail of booze, cheap aftershave, excitement and, simmering beneath, an undertone of menace. They'd all reached that stage of the evening where they were willing something to happen. Whether I liked it or not, I'd become the night's star attraction.

Once again I said to myself, *I don't want any part of this*, but I couldn't make out a single escape route that wouldn't also see me losing face. Which, at the time, was far more important to me than it should have been. So the contest began. We both strained for a bit. Or at least as much as two men who could only just about see straight could manage. But neither of our arms budged. Stalemate. We both swigged our drinks, and I experienced a brief moment of relief. I thought that the ordeal was over.

The relief lasted until someone else shouted, 'Left arms!' *You must be fucking kidding me*. Still, I couldn't bring myself to walk away. We used different arms, but we got the same result. My opponent was ecstatic, his whole face filled with a gleeful malice. 'You and your fucking muscles aren't worth shit.' He pointed at me in delight and got up. For a second I even thought he was going to start dancing.

That's when my mate leant over and, like a devil sitting on my shoulder, said into my ear, 'Are you going to let him get away with that?'

I'd not thought anything of it. I wasn't that bothered, he was just another twat in a club full of twats. If I was going to start on everyone who said something stupid to me, I'd be scrapping all night. All I wanted was for this nonsense to be over. At least, so I told myself.

But my mate's words went straight to the worst bit of me. Why was I going to let this skinny fuck take the piss? Seconds ago I couldn't have cared less. Now I was fucking adamant that he was *not* going to get away with it. The next thing I remember is grabbing this guy and sticking him one. The whole place erupted. Glasses got smashed, tables and chairs skittered over, blood and beer started to seep into the carpet. Before I knew it I was fighting with the doormen and on my way to being kicked out, along with the lad I'd been arm-wrestling with. There was a bit more scuffling under the neon lights of the club's car park, then the police turned up and I was arrested.

I thought that I was so far from that headspace, that me and my mate were just two drunk fuckers having a joke and a laugh. But all it needed was one seed of doubt and everything changed. In the blink of an eye I'd returned to being the sort of person I didn't want to be. How was any of this going to help me become the best version of myself? The only place it led to was waking up in a prison cell with a bruised face, a sickening hangover and the knowledge that I was going to have to explain to Emilie why I'd fucked up again.

I WISH I'D had the confidence to say No. I wish I'd believed in myself more, realised that I was better than what I was about to do. But at that time in my life I thought I had a reputation to uphold. The problem was that it was really somebody else's reputation. That wasn't me. It was just the person I felt I needed to be to survive in that social environment. And it was also holding me back. I thought I was just wearing a costume, when actually I was wearing a straitjacket.

I guarantee that these words will resonate with people. Because there are so many people who know that they're living lives that aren't true to themselves. I think there are probably even more who have an inkling of it. They're working jobs they don't like, or hanging around with people they know aren't good for them. They can feel that their clothes don't fit – they're too tight in some places, too baggy in others – but they haven't quite worked out how to escape that existence.

You'll never be successful wearing somebody else's clothes. Everything will always be a compromise. Instead, you've got to find a way of living an authentic life. An authentic life is one in which you've stopped lying to yourself and others. You're proud of who you are and what you stand for. When you live an authentic life you follow your own instincts rather than squashing yourself to fit somebody else's expectations.

And when you know yourself, when you're true to yourself, you'll find it far easier to be decisive. So many people spend their lives wracked by indecision. They're dizzy with uncertainty. The main reason for this is that they don't have a clear sense of who they are or what their priorities should be. They second-guess themselves. Or they spend too much time worrying what other people might think. Somewhere along the way they've got muddled. Every choice now becomes far tougher than it needs to be. They're like badly tuned radios. Instead of one clear channel, their heads are full of fuzzy voices and distorted songs.

When you lead an authentic life you'll be happier, more fulfilled and more confident, because you're the author of your own existence. Only one person should be writing the story of your life: you.

THE ONLY OPINION THAT MATTERS

There are seven billion opinions on the planet. Yours is the only one that should matter.

These days I'm so sure of who I am. Whatever people say about me, I've got foundations I know I can fall back on.

But that hasn't always been the case. When I let my mate wind me up on that night out in Essex it was because I wasn't confident enough to say, 'No, that's not who I am.' I was too susceptible to external pressure, I cared too much about what others thought.

That's not surprising. It can sometimes feel as if the easiest, most rewarding way of existing is to conform to what other people want from us – whether they're troublemakers looking to play on your worst instincts, or do-gooders who claim they know what's best for you.

I can see the attraction of a sense of belonging. But you should never pursue that at the expense of surrendering your integrity. That's what I did briefly in the Paras. I was so desperate to be accepted by the other soldiers on their terms that my behaviour sometimes betrayed the things I value, such as respecting other people and standing up for yourself.

Confident people are people who are able to think differently. They don't mind being the one who goes against the crowd, because for them the price of surrendering their authenticity is higher than whatever brief reward comes from merely fitting in. And yet so much about the way we're expected to live seems designed to keep us in rigid, blinkered lanes that limit us both physically and psychologically and restrict the way we think. It's almost as if the people in charge don't want us to build the confidence that comes with trying new things, new ways of being.

Instead we live lives that are forced upon us. The psychological price to pay for living the 'wrong' life is immense. Think of all those people who became lawyers or went into the City because their parents expected them to, and who ended up having a fuck-off midlife crisis when they hit forty. I got married the first time round – to Hayley – because my personality at the time was of somebody who just went along with things. I thought being able to just go with the flow was really important. But I realised that choosing the easy route, being a yes man, just doesn't work. People can end up eating shit their whole lives.

So many of us are square pegs rammed into round holes. You'll either remain like that for the rest of your existence, saying, 'Tell me what to do,' 'Tell me what to say,' which the majority of people end up doing, or you'll move from hole to hole until you find the one that fits. You'll forge your own path rather than following the route others try to lay out for you. You've got to take a stance, you've got to stay true to who you are. When your moral compass swings violently away from true north, then you have to reset it.

If you live a life that's true to yourself, if you can strip away all the bullshit and exist on your own terms, you'll live a happy, positive life. It's something that can't be bought or faked. That's why I refuse to conform.

THERE IS NO NORMAL

People use the idea of 'normal' to try to make you fit their agendas. They pretend that the idea has some sort of objective reality. The implication is that if you don't comply, there's something wrong with you. 'Oh, a normal person would be trying to get this sort of job,' or 'A normal person wouldn't do that.'

But it's not a problem if you don't fit in with what other people consider 'normal'. In fact, I'm not sure I even know what normal means. What is normal? It's something we don't think about enough. Instead, we just dumbly accept other people's definition of normal and contort ourselves to try to fit in. And yet in truth, everybody's normal is different. Normal for me is jumping out of a helicopter or climbing Mount Everest. Normal for you will be something else entirely. Normal in the Paras was drinking warm piss out of a desert boot. Whatever anybody else tries to tell you, remember that THERE. IS. NO. NORMAL.

Don't let anybody use the idea of what is and isn't 'normal' to bully you into being somebody, or doing something, you're uncomfortable with.

BUILD A CASTLE

Now that I've reached the point where I'm much clearer about who I am and what my values are, I'm extra-determined to hold tight to that identity. I don't want to waste the effort I've put in to finding out who I am, and I don't want that identity to be diluted or diverted by other people.

Of course, we all have to jump through hoops or sing from a shared hymn sheet from time to time. It's unavoidable unless you're somebody like Anthony Joshua, Conor McGregor or LeBron James and have what I like to call 'fuck-you money'. They can say whatever they like without having to think about the consequences. Their wealth makes them un-cancellable: 'You want to try to ruin my career? Fine, I'll fuck off to a superyacht in the Maldives.'

Build a castle around your authentic self. Resist the people who will try to pigeonhole you or scrub off your rough edges. You know what's best for you. I've spent too much time letting other people and external situations rule my life. It's brought me to the psychological brink.

If someone comes to me with an idea and at any point it makes me think, *Why would I do this?* then I'm not going to go any further. I don't care how amazing a sponsorship deal it is, or how big a TV platform. I'd be willing to lose *everything* in order to stay true to myself. Because if the price is living a false life, then what really would I be gaining?

Don't you hate that feeling of going along with something that you know is wrong because somebody has said it's the best thing for you to do? All you want to scream is 'Stop, stop, stop.' But you carry on, and before you know it you've been transformed into somebody you barely recognise.

If another person is trying to guide you – and it might well be for the best of reasons – and that first footstep doesn't feel right to you, then do not start on that path. Every step you take after that will be a step away from the real you.

I'm really happy for people to say try this, try that. I'll step into most corridors. But as soon as it doesn't feel right,

I'll stop. Being confident enough to say, 'No, that's not who I am' isn't easy – actually, it's hard as hell – and yet it's so important.

You say to yourself, 'That person has put in all this work', or 'They seem to know what they're doing,' and you override all of your own concerns and agree. It's nice to be a go-along and get-along sort. So you agree to the course of action they suggest and then at some point you find yourself stuck. I've been there, regretted that. Because the further away you walk away from that original flame that inspired you, the more likely it is to burn out. I hear it all the time when I do corporate talks. Men and women come up to me and tell me that their flame was extinguished ages ago. I tell them to go back to the first time it began to flicker and sputter.

'But that was years ago!' they reply.

'Can't you take what embers are left from the old flame, and use them to start a new one? You've changed, your ideas and priorities have shifted, but the fact alone that we're talking means that something must be left,' I'll say.

Still, although it's possible to rekindle that spark, how much better to never let the flame go out at all.

That's why I try to teach my kids to question everything. I don't want them to fall unthinkingly into the grind of everyday life. They will get stuff wrong, or someone will turn around and say, 'Well, we actually do this for a reason.' Great, they'll learn something either way!

LIVE BY YOUR STANDARDS, NOT OTHER PEOPLE'S

There are far fewer objective measures of success and failure than you might think. What might be a dismal failure to one person would be a dazzling success to me. The opposite is also true. If you do something that other people go wild about, but you know deep down that you've fallen short of the standards you expect of yourself, don't take the easy route of basking in their acclaim.

Never forget that. If you live life according to other people's definition of success you will *never* be happy. When you do that, you'll be a slave to those external, bullshit injunctions that are forced upon us all: you have to have this job or this salary by this age, or by the time you're this age you should have a family and kids.

And society is fickle. There are always going to be fads. What we find acceptable now will be condemned in the future. That makes it all the more important to hold tight to our values and avoid getting swayed by here-today-gone-to-morrow fashions.

If you look at the world from the outside in, you'll always be chasing something. If you look at in from the inside out, you'll be doing what you want to do and what you feel is right, not trying to please others. Listen to your internal voice. When you're judging yourself by your own standards, not other people's, there's very little that can touch you. People can say what they want about me. I don't care, because I know that it's all words. It's all fucking nonsense. People can tarnish my name until the cows come home. Let them. Those that know me know the truth about me. That's what's important. I don't give a shit what some journalist slapping at his laptop keys because he's literally got *nothing* better to write about says. There are bigger things to worry about in this world than whether somebody doesn't like one of my Instagram posts or is upset by something I've said on *SAS: Who Dares Wins*.

If you're confident in your inner self, if you work hard to stay authentic, then it doesn't matter what anybody else says. You'll know that you're living a life that matches the standards you have set for yourself.

And, do you know what? It's fine not to be everybody's cup of tea. You don't have to make everyone like you. You don't have to seek the approval of every human being on the planet. The day I understood that was the day I began to feel a lot more free.

ESCAPE THE ANT COLONY

One of the most insidious aspect of society at the moment is people's desire to try to deny some of the most significant elements in our make-up.

Look at what's in our DNA as human beings. Once upon a time we were far from the top of the food chain, but over thousands of years we've fought our way to get there. The significant word is 'fought'. Fighting is innate to us. And I think it's dangerous to suppress our desire for conflict. There's a beast inside us that needs to be exercised, otherwise it will tear us apart from the inside out.

I sometimes think we're becoming like those sad, caged lions you sometimes see in zoos. Mangy fur, listless and weakened – because they're trapped and their nature has been squashed – but still essentially vicious. We're losing our identities because our own fighting instinct has been suppressed. Instead of doing all the things that are innate to us, we're stuck inside offices listening to dickheads telling us off because we haven't sent the right email at the right time to the right person. 'Keep your mouth shut and your head down, and if you're a good boy we'll give you a pension contribution.' Fuck. That.

If you don't want all of the aggression and anger that lie within us to build up and turn ugly, it's important to exercise the beast within. Yet society doesn't cater for that process anymore. It doesn't offer us the chance to go out there and peel those layers off, find ways to push ourselves to your limits and do the things that are so out of place in our antiseptic existence, activities with an edge that get the adrenaline pumping through your system and make serious demands on both your body and your mind. Of course, I'm not suggesting that you get in touch with your inner Viking and go and pillage some monasteries, fun as that might be. The activities have to be controlled and constructive.

That's why I think stuff like martial arts can literally be a life-saver. It's not just that something such as Brazilian jiu-jitsu teaches you about teamwork and helps you build your confidence. It also provides the sort of outlet that doesn't appear much anymore. Do what you can to escape from the ant colony our life has become.

GREAT MINDS DON'T THINK ALIKE

I don't see race, just as I don't see gender or religion. All I'm interested in is: are you a cunt or not? If you are, I'm probably not going to get on with you. But I don't give a fuck about the colour of your skin. I want to judge everybody on their own merits, so why would I have any preconceptions or prejudices about their ethnic background? It doesn't make sense.

We should be focusing on the individual, not their ethnicity or faith. Reducing somebody to their background has a flattening effect. We see people as a Muslim or a Nigerian before we see them as a unique human being. That way of thinking actually ends up giving prejudice a helping hand. In fact, I think we're so caught up in thinking about colour and race in the UK that it has ended up dividing us.

I'm not on anybody's side, because as soon as you support one side, you're automatically set against the other. And when it comes to navigating the differences between us, I believe in common sense. Good manners. Respect. Kindness. Treating other people in the way you'd like to be treated yourself. The simplest things there are, but it can feel now as if there's no space for them. I don't care what race, gender or religion you are – I'll respect you. I'll use whatever pronouns or names you want me to. I'm not going to say anything derogatory about your beliefs. It's so simple that I don't understand why we need to complicate it with so much PC bullshit. Life is complicated. We're very complicated beings. Why *add* any more complexity to that mix? Why reduce interactions with other human beings to a series of tick boxes? Sometimes it feels as if we're being tested. It's like there are people just waiting for others to use the wrong word in the wrong place at the wrong time.

All I ask is that you show me the same respect that I'd show you. I don't see why some people find that so hard to do. When I tell people that my wife loves being a full-time mum (looking after four kids while I'm off gallivanting: the hardest job in the world), they'll sometimes say, 'She needs to get with the times.'

What? I'd never tell you how to organise your family life. As long as what I'm doing isn't hurting anybody, why the fuck do you think you have the right to judge me? Everyone makes their own choices about how to live. You don't have to agree with those choices, but you do have to respect them. Why do we all have to be the same?

I love talking to new people. Finding out about how other people live their lives, working out what makes them tick, learning about their experiences. I love all of that. And that's why I welcome diversity. For me, diversity has nothing to do with skin colour. It's about having a diverse way of thinking. If you're from an African country with a different culture, you'll have different perspectives to me. Great! It means that when confronted by a challenge, we've got more than one way of approaching it. Diversity – whether it's about education or life experience – is an amazing strength for a team.

SPEAK FREELY BUT KINDLY

I've got a free mind. You can take literally everything you want away from me, but I'll always have the way I think. It's important to me to express myself, whether that's standing up for my own values, or stepping in to support other people.

That's what's earned me a reputation for being outspoken. I don't go out to offend. I go out to tell the truth. Sometimes that works out, sometimes it doesn't. The irony is that I became famous because I speak my mind, because I'm true to myself, but the longer I go on, and the higher I get, the greater the pressure has become for me to shut up and conform. Work that one out!

I know people who are afraid of expressing themselves because if they don't they won't be able to put food on their family's table. It's a career-stopper. Why risk a life you've spent ten, fifteen years carefully putting together? But that doesn't fucking rub with me. It's dangerous to bottle stuff up. If you spend your whole time suppressing your voice, you'll begin to lose sight of who you are.

We're told to express ourselves, and then when we do exactly that, we get told off for expressing ourselves in the wrong way. Is it any wonder that so many people are throwing their hands up and asking, 'Well, who the *fuck* am I?'

As long as your motives are good, as long as you're not deliberately trying to hurt people, or make them feel uncomfortable, then you shouldn't feel afraid of speaking up.

LESSONS

Don't be a square peg in a round hole. When you suppress your instincts and personality to fit somebody else's agenda, you'll end up living a crushed, unsatisfying life.

Your authentic self is precious. Guard it fiercely. Resist any attempts to make you go down paths you know aren't right for you. There's only one person whose opinion should matter: you.

'Normal' is a concept designed to make us conform. You should never forget that everybody's 'normal' is different. So don't let anybody persuade you otherwise.

Pay attention to individuals, not identities. You should never make assumptions about somebody based on the colour of their skin, their gender or the faith they follow. Look past these to the person behind them.

If you demand respect, you've got to give it too. If I need to explain this to you, I don't think I can help you.

CHAPTER 4

LIVE YOUR LIFE RIGHT

How to build a healthy, balanced lifestyle that can become the foundation for building a better you.

FILMING MUTINY LEFT me physically and mentally fucked. Along with eight volunteers I'd recreated the savage 4,000-mile journey from Tonga to Timor that Captain Bligh and his crew had undertaken over two hundred years earlier, in 1789. They'd been forced into that ordeal by mutineers aboard their ship, the HMS *Bounty*; we'd *chosen* to do it. Our desire to make the experience as authentic as possible meant that we were in a replica of their tiny wooden boat. We also used the diary that Bligh had kept during his voyage as a survival handbook.

This all made for great TV, but it left us completely exposed to the cruel heat and furious storms of the South Pacific. We navigated using charts, refused waterproof clothing and struggled on a meagre diet of dry biscuits and increasingly stale water. All of this was exacerbated by the sometimes violent tensions that emerged among our crew, which actually led to one of them having to leave our boat.

It was the closest thing to hell I've ever experienced.

I remember how the first thing I did after I stumbled ashore off the boat in Timor was to call Emilie, who had been seven months pregnant when I'd left for Tonga two months earlier.

'Great,' she said, 'I'm glad you're safe. But don't forget I'm due to give birth today.'

I was meant to go to Bali for five days of R&R. They even had a psychologist lined up. 'I can't,' I told them. 'I've got to get on the next flight home.'

After signing a waiver to confirm I was ignoring literally every piece of advice they'd given me, I was booked onto a flight the following morning. I had to get back.

We'd filmed the first series of SAS: *Who Dares Wins* not long before *Mutiny*, but it hadn't yet been broadcast. Nobody knew whether it would be a hit; it was just a programme that Channel 4 had a few hopes for. So I was in cattle class, with an aisle seat. For the first few minutes I shifted around trying to get comfortable. I still wasn't used to the changes that the past weeks had wrought on my body and mind. The lifting of the psychological burden of being responsible for the well-being and morale of the other guys, which had pressed down on me for so long, had initially been an extraordinary relief. And yet I realised that part of that continued to linger inside me. I would have moments when I suddenly found myself gripped by an intense worry – about the water that became undrinkable, or one of the contestants' hostility – as if it was still up to me to sort these things out.

At the same time, there was so much that had occurred during the previous months that I could barely recall. I think that while at sea I'd been so intent on getting by on a tiny amount of food and water that I'd lost the ability to form memories. Instead my body acted as a kind of record of what I'd been through.

I still had livid marks on my leg and foot from where I'd accidentally hacked myself open with an axe. The improvised stitches had held, but the wounds hurt and looked ugly. Most of all I was tired. I'd given everything I could, day after day. The sun had been relentless, sapping energy from me that I lacked the resources to replace. My eyes were sunken in my skull, and every time I shifted in my seat I was given another reminder of all the muscle mass that had wasted away. When we were weighed, I was horrified to discover that I'd lost four stone. The photographs I took that day are still shocking.

I realised that I'd sustained a heavy psychological toll too. The first time I picked up an iPhone in two months I stared blankly at the screen – I'd completely forgotten how it worked. I didn't know how to scroll through it, and I was *amazed* that it didn't have a keypad. I was pawing at it like a monkey, my mind completely blown. It had become so much part of my life before I'd got on that boat – in my pocket 24/7 – that I'd come to take it for granted.

It wasn't the only thing that I'd relied on without ever really appreciating it. For years I'd been accustomed to feeling strong, both mentally and physically. I was proud of this – it was the bedrock of all that I'd achieved. Now it seemed as if my strength had gone. I felt vulnerable and weak, and although I was exhausted I was gripped by a restlessness that meant I couldn't get to sleep, no matter how hard I tried.

Eventually, just as a little kid toddled past my feet, I nearly managed to drift off. But somehow the child's light, unsteady steps became distorted in my ragged mind. I grabbed hold of him and started screaming hoarsely into his face. 'What are you doing on my boat? What are you doing on my boat?' Then I stopped, abruptly. I was appalled by what I'd just done. I cannot imagine how that poor lad must have felt. My hair was straggly, my face was gaunt – I must have looked like a starving and crazy half-man, half-wolf. The boy looked at me for a single, shocked second, then dissolved into tears.

I watched him run off to the other end of the plane, then decided to follow him to try to resolve the situation. I caught up with him just as he reached his mum, who had clearly decided there was some connection between her weeping son and the mad-looking fucker who had suddenly materialised by her seat.

'What happened?' she asked me, her expression a mix of suspicion and concern. I tried to explain. Most of all I apologised. Initially my story must have sounded pretty unbelievable. But she was great. I think she understood what kind of a state I was in, and how horrified I was by what had happened. She knew that I meant no harm.

'Don't worry,' she reassured me, 'and thanks for coming over and letting me know. Just promise me you'll get some rest.'

I WISH I could have kept my promise to her. It's not that I didn't want to put my feet up. But I had a wife and three kids waiting for me, with a baby scheduled to arrive at any minute. Emilie, especially, who had been almost all on her own for two months, was in a bad way. Her concerns over the baby growing inside her had been mounting, and I hadn't been there for her to confide in or to reassure her. I knew that I would have to step up as soon as I walked through the door.

Emilie ended up having an emergency C-section. I'd made my journey; it was Emilie and Bligh's that mattered now. The more of their stress and pressure I could take on board the better. Plus, there were three other kids who still needed to be fed, entertained and put to bed. I didn't have time to think about myself or how I felt. When, exactly, was I supposed to have a rest? Before I knew it I was knee-deep in the routines familiar to anybody with a young family: school runs, changing nappies, intervening in confusing arguments about the precise ownership of a particular toy.

The same was true after Everest. I'd lost a lot of weight that time too, again through muscle deterioration. I was snowblind in one eye and my feet were fucked. My family was even bigger then, the kids older and more demanding. I just had to trust the process.

On neither occasion could I afford to dwell on 'recovery'. My mind was full of other questions: 'Where's the next job?', 'How can I provide for my family?'

And yet both times I quickly got better.

WHAT MADE THE difference after coming back from my exertions on the other side of the planet wasn't a micro-targeted recovery programme or even taking an extended break. It was simply the fact of being reabsorbed into the daily rhythms of family life.

After *Mutiny*, I resumed the lifestyle I'd had to abandon when I left for Tonga. I went to bed early and got a full night's sleep – although to begin with I'd sometimes wake up with a start during the night, convinced I was still on that fucking boat. Even during the day I realised that I'd become so used to the ship's motion on the waves that there were times when I was convinced I could still feel its rise and fall within me.

I ate a great deal – I was no longer going to be subjected to the same rations as on the boat – but it was always the sort of healthy yet unremarkable meals that were part of my family's normal diet. There weren't any magic juices or secret ingredients. I didn't pop recovery pills. And after a while I was back to eating a more sensible amount.

My kidneys and liver had been given a pounding by the long, hot days with so little water. Again, the solution was simple. You don't need to be a nutritionist to know that I just had to rehydrate.

I started to exercise again, tentatively at first. But I knew it was important to get back into the habit of raising my heartbeat, and I felt an enormous benefit from the simple process of feeling my body being flooded with oxygen and endorphins.

And I was always, always busy. Being among my family meant that I could focus on people other than myself. If you sit there telling yourself how awfully tired you are you're probably not going to stop feeling tired anytime soon. Don't let yourself languish. Life goes on. There isn't time to stop that wheel from turning.

What all of this taught me was that people overthink recovery. Your body is fucking amazing – you just need to trust that it will do the work you need it to do. It will heal. Think about how it repairs itself after a cut or a broken bone. It performs miracles on our behalf every single day, and yet we take it for granted. If you're injured, then you clearly need to take the right steps to make sure it heals. Otherwise, your body will replenish itself.

While people might overthink recovery, I'd maintain they also underthink and therefore underrate the importance of lifestyle. Recovery isn't a once-in-a-month activity. It's a life-style. It should be a continuous process, not a sticking plaster you occasionally remember to slap on. And at the heart of a healthy lifestyle should be the understanding that a healthy body comes hand in hand with having a healthy mind. You can't have one without the other. What you put in your body, how much sleep you get, the effort you invest in your mental well-being, the people you surround yourself with – they're all connected.

You might be in brilliant mental shape, but if your body starts to deteriorate it will affect your psychological well-being. If you're physically fit but you're not in a great mental headspace, then you're always going to be vulnerable. You can train and train for year after year, yet as soon as you find yourself exposed to a setback you'll break. None of that muscle will be able to save you. You'll fall straight through that trapdoor.

I'm living proof of this interconnection. I know that when my body gets weak – whether it's because I've not been eating right, or not getting enough sleep or exercise – my mind gets dragged down. My thinking isn't quite as sharp, my mood is lower. Resilience isn't just a mental quality. How are you going to withstand heavy emotional pressure if you're knackered because you've been going to bed at 2 a.m. every night and stuffing your face with fast food?

That's why I make sure my lifestyle is right. Have a good routine, listen to your body, eat sensibly, take the time to give your body and brain a workout, get a proper night's sleep and don't abuse your body by getting pissed all the time. It's no more complex than that. If you follow a healthy, balanced lifestyle, you're creating the most amazing foundation for your ambitions – whether that's because you want to get the absolute maximum out of yourself or simply want to maintain a decent level of mental and physical fitness.

THE POWER OF ROUTINE

I want to maximise my day. But saying this isn't enough by itself; you have to create the conditions in which it can happen.

The best method is having a good routine. Routines are the foundation on which the rest of your lifestyle can be built. When you have discipline and structure in your life, motivation becomes far easier. You're not fighting against the day – you're working with it. When you live a baggy, unstructured life, you'll always be reacting to situations. You'll be stressed and anxious because you're forever one step behind. Why would you do that to yourself?

If you create a basic framework for the day, everything becomes more straightforward. You don't have to make as many choices, because you already know what you're going to be doing. It makes it easier both to maintain good habits – like exercise and eating right – and to drop bad ones. And it helps you prioritise: you can determine in advance what your most important tasks are, and then give yourself time and space to complete them. You're not juggling everything, trying to work out which job to start first. That's why many people who don't have a routine will tell you that before the end of the morning they're already feeling stressed, anxious or overwhelmed.

I'm not saying you should have a complex, colour-coded plan that allocates a particular activity for every minute. But I do think you should have a structure that allows you to be proactive and shape the day. I'm like anybody else – I often feel as if there aren't enough hours in the day. I wish I had more time to work out, more time to recover, more time to work. I definitely wish I had more time with my family. Yet when you've got a routine, you're better able to balance all the different parts of your life.

Of course, nothing's set in stone. There will be weeks where I work eighty, ninety hours, and inevitably that eats into the other parts of my life. But I know it's not sustainable. You can't live your life at that pace forever.

The most important thing is to keep it simple. Ask yourself: what do I need to make my day run as well as it possibly can? What can I prepare in advance to prevent unnecessary hassle?

*   *   *

A TYPICAL DAY for me unfolds a bit like this:

I wake up at 6 a.m. First thing I do is have a glass of water. I think this kickstarts your body. Then I get up and let the dog out. Next I wake the kids up ready for school. They'll all have folded their uniform the night before. I don't want them getting up in the morning tearing about in a panic because they don't know where their school blazer is.

After Emilie wakes up, we have breakfast. I have a smoothie and some fruit. Once the whaaaa of the machine has died down I look around to check that everyone is OK. Have they started the day in a positive headspace? If any of the kids is looking miserable I'll play a little joke on them, give them a kiss or a cuddle.

At 7.30 Emilie takes them off to school, and I go to the gym for half an hour. I might go on the treadmill, the cross-trainer or the rowing machine. Having a balanced lifestyle doesn't mean living in the gym. I certainly don't. I can't spend hours on end in there because I've got an extremely busy work life and five kids, so half an hour a day is enough. And half an hour is sustainable. I know I can fit that into my schedule. If work or whatever limits the amount of time I have to exercise, I'll always prioritise cardiovascular train-ing over muscle-building. You've got to keep your heart pumping, your lungs open and your brain firing. Everything else follows from that.

Once I've showered, it's time to work. I find it easy to throw myself into whatever I've got in front of me – whether it's a catch-up with my publishers, an interview with a journalist or a business meeting – because I've already made a dynamic start. All the small stages I've mentioned so far might seem insignificant in themselves, but I see them as the foundation of my day. They're a series of building blocks that help me get my mindset right. If you begin each morning by dithering or making excuses, then you'll stay in that frame of mind until it's too late to actually get anything done. But if you start the day with purpose and direction, you'll create a momentum that allows you to ignore all the nagging voices that try to disrupt your progress: 'I haven't got the energy for this right now,' 'I had a shit night's sleep,' 'It looks way too complicated.' Everyone is tempted by these cop-outs, but when you've got a good routine it's far easier to resist them.

I try to have a light lunch like a chicken wrap or an omelette – I don't want to feel bloated all afternoon.

Afterwards, I might drive into London for meetings in the afternoon or there might be a photoshoot. Either way, I make sure I'm back in time for an early dinner with the whole family. I want to eat with my children. I see it as the most important meal of the day. Once it's in your system, your body has the whole night to absorb and digest it.

We eat sensibly, stuff like salmon, rockfish, sole, chicken, quinoa, potatoes, lots of vegetables. But we're not in the business of punishing ourselves. I've got kids, so of course I eat chocolate and cake. Like everything else, eating is about balance.

I put Priseïs and Bligh to bed between 6 and 6.30. I'll read them a story, and once they're asleep I'll hit the gym again for half an hour of circuits. As before, it's something I can easily slot into my schedule without disrupting anything else.

After this I get to spend the rest of the evening with Emilie. That time together is precious. We can relax and watch TV, but it also gives us the chance to share and process our experiences of the day. We can talk about what's happened to us both or to the kids. Most importantly, we can talk through any problems. It's really important to metabolise anything difficult that might have cropped up. It's much better to resolve – or at least start to address – those things before you try to sleep.

ALL OF THIS has become an integral part of my life. When I have to skip any element I feel a very strong sense of something missing. It's a bit like when your kids stay the night somewhere else. The whole house feels empty and strange, and I get grumpy and out of sorts.

What I've just described is what works for me and my family. You'll have different priorities and time pressures. You might have a job that means you need to be in an office from 9 to 5 or you might work shift patterns that require you to sleep during the day. I can't tell you exactly how to arrange your existence; that's something you'll need to sort out. But it will be worth the effort.

GET YOUR BLOOD PUMPING

Exercise is a crucial part of my life – I wouldn't be able to function without it. It's a good way of getting out of your own head and it's the surest way of getting that rush of endorphins, the unmistakable feeling in your limbs telling you that you've pushed them hard.

When I head out on a run or go to the gym, I'm making sure that blood is flowing around my body, my arteries aren't blocked and that there's enough oxygen in my brain to ensure that I can keep on thinking clearly. Afterwards I feel flexible, elasticated, I can feel my blood pumping, I feel *alive*.

Clearly I need to be physically fit to do many aspects of my job. *SAS: Who Dares Wins* is as demanding of my energy as it is of the recruits', because I'm with them every step of the way. If I turned up looking like a fat fuck I'd not only struggle to assert my authority, I'd also find it very hard to keep up. More generally, I'm a very busy person. I've got a wide range of personal and professional commitment, so I need the energy that being in good shape provides to be able to do all of those things to the standards I expect of myself.

Plus, looking ahead, I know that the better condition I keep my body in, the longer I'll be able to lead an active, happy life.

I want to live as long as I can. I want to still be here when I'm 150. Another 110 years on this planet – that excites the shit out of me. You can buy time by looking after yourself: eating healthily, being positive, and not dragging unnecessary stress and anxiety onto your shoulders. But exercise is always going to be the thing that makes the most difference.

When you exercise regularly, you reduce your risk of developing chronic conditions such as diabetes and heart disease, and even some cancers.

There's also a symbiotic relationship between the exercise I take and my mental state. It improves my mood and the quality of my sleep. The mere fact of exercising makes me feel better about myself.

Find something that you enjoy, otherwise you'll find it really hard to stick at it. It doesn't matter what you choose – dancing, football, cycling, climbing, swimming – as long as you're doing something energetic enough that you can feel your heart beating faster, your breathing getting quicker and your body feeling warmer.

The other crucial aspect is that it must be something you can easily fit into your schedule. The most important question you should ask yourself is not 'What *should* I do?', it's 'What *can* I do?' What you have to ensure is that the exercise you take is compatible with the rest of your life. It's impractical to always be disappearing on training camps. It's easy to incorporate short bursts into your day-to-day routine: perhaps you can get up half an hour earlier than normal to go for a run; or you could cycle to work instead of getting the bus. If you can get up a sweat playing with your kids in the garden, or doing exercise videos in your kitchen, then brilliant!

If you exercise like this every day that you can, you'll end up an extremely fit person. And that's all without beasting yourself. There's no need to hurry when it comes to fitness. Do not fucking rush. Why do you *need* to lose weight in six weeks? I'm not saying that you won't lose the pounds you want to get rid of in that time. You probably will. But I'd be willing to lay a fair-sized bet that they'll pile back on pretty quickly afterwards. That's because this type of exercise isn't part of your life. It's not sustainable. Programmes have their place. But they're always going to be a short-term fix.

EXERCISE YOUR BRAIN

Some people rely on their physical fitness to maintain their psychological strength. They believe that keeping their blood pumping is enough by itself to maintain their mental well-being. It's certainly a start, but no more.

The good news is that you can exercise your brain just as you can any other part of your body. Technically speaking, the brain is an organ, just like the liver or the lungs. But I find it useful to think about it as if it's a muscle. That's why

I work on it every day, by challenging negativity, putting myself in difficult situations.

In addition to the techniques for growing your mental fitness I discuss in Chapter 12 on resilience, Chapter 2 on confidence and Chapter 11 on controlling your emotions, there's so much you can do too. Just being out and about in the world has its own value. If you're connecting with other human beings, going to unfamiliar places, doing unfamiliar things, then you're making your brain work. Take up fresh hobbies and practise new skills. Learn to speak a new language or play a musical instrument. Read stimulating books. Again, as with physical exercise, these activities must be things that you can fit comfortably into your day-to-day existence. They have to be sustainable too, things you're happy to do repeatedly over a long period of time rather than just in short bursts.

If you're constantly asking your brain to do new things, if you challenge it every day, you'll be helping it to grow and stay healthy.

THE WINDOW

I believe that there's a window – between the ages of twenty-five and fifty – when we enjoy supreme physical health, when our body is designed to be at the peak of its endurance. There's a reason why the lads who pass Selection are at the back end of their twenties or into their early thirties. Only a handful ever get into the Special Forces younger than that. Your physical and mental endurance only really kicks in properly after you've passed twenty-five.

But once you pass fifty you're going to be more and more plagued by little niggles, and your body will take longer to recover.

It's during this window that you should set up the good habits that will stand you in good stead in the years to come. The earlier you make exercise, eating and drinking right, and sleeping properly a part of your life, the easier it will be to sustain them. It's so much harder to start all these things from scratch once you've crossed into middle age, and your body doesn't respond as easily.

A lot of people get to their fifties without ever really having taken much exercise. Then they find themselves carrying too much weight or they have a health scare. Although it's very rare that it's too late to get yourself in shape, it's far harder to get going when you've hit your fifties. It's like getting an oil tanker to turn. You don't want to be in the position where you're asking yourself, 'Why didn't I start this in my twenties?' Prevention is far easier and far more effective than any cure will ever be.

Almost all of us are given this window of opportunity – make sure you don't waste it.

LISTEN TO YOUR BODY

The same lifestyle isn't going to work for everybody, obviously. We all have different physiques, different demands on our time and different priorities. You can learn from what others do – in fact you should always be alert to the gems you can grab from other people, but you shouldn't be looking to copy them slavishly.

In any case, you already possess the best possible guide to what you need to live a good lifestyle: your very own body. Your body is in constant communication with you. It sends you an unceasing flood of information right through the day, letting you know when something is wrong, when you're hungry or when you need to sleep. Yet a lot of the time you ignore what it's trying to tell you.

Learning to listen to my body and its demands is one of the best things I've ever done. It was by listening to my body that I recovered after the exertions of the *Mutiny* experience. When it told me I was hungry, I ate; when it told me I was thirsty, I drank; when it told me it was tired, I slept.

As far as your day-to-day lifestyle goes, it's another situation where trial and error is absolutely key to working out how you function at your best. You hold all the answers already, it's just that they won't necessarily come immediately. You have to keep watching and learning.

For instance, you might find that you feel at your best after you've eaten a particular food at a particular time or that if you go to bed after midnight you feel shit the next day. You know when you're slightly overweight or when you get a little bit out of breath climbing up a flight of stairs. Some people feel stronger when they're carrying a bit more weight, while others feel more energetic when they're lighter.

All of this is your body sending out signals. It *wants* to be heard, so make a note of that. When you've done so, it's up to you to have the discipline needed to address what your body has demanded. I'll *know* when I'm a bit out of shape or I need to lose two or three kilos, because I'm attuned to my body. There's nothing, almost nothing, better than that moment on a winter's morning when you open the door to let the dog out and you can fill your lungs with a huge gulp of air. But if there's ever a moment when I cough or my lungs just don't fill up quite right, I'll get pissed off. 'Right, fucking hell, I need to up my ante.' That's my prompt to do forty-five minutes in the gym instead of just thirty.

I've found that the messages your body sends you about your general physical well-being are simple, and so are the solutions. If you're hanging out of your arse every time you go from the kitchen to your bedroom, you don't need a complex exercise programme; you just need to get your body moving. Start swimming, cycling or running. If you decide on running, for example, begin by smashing out 3K in the mornings; then when you're feeling fitter, up it to 5K. After a year, you might be doing 10K.

(One thing to note: if you're upping your exercise levels on your own like this, be more attentive to how you feel than if you're on an off-the-peg schedule. Don't stretch yourself too much too soon. Take it slowly, otherwise you'll run the risk of injuring yourself. Make a small, incremental increase, then see how your body responds. If you're feeling OK, build it up again.)

Food is another area where we're out of touch with our body's demands and needs. It's so easy to subscribe to the idea that even if all the other diets you've tried have failed, there's one that will work for you. That's bollocks. There's no one-size-fits-all solution to our often complex relation-ship with food. Nobody's lurking out there with a magic wand just waiting to tell you exactly how many grams of carbohydrates you're allowed at any given sitting. It's up to you to do the work.

We often eat because we can, not because we need to. A lot of the time we overeat and overdrink out of sheer bore-dom. It almost becomes a reflex – our mind wanders and almost before we know it we've eaten that sandwich or downed that Coke. On other occasions, our overeating is a response to emotional rather than physical cues. We get sad, so we fill ourselves with junk because we think it will make us feel better. And, of course, the opposite generally happens.

Instead of feeling happier we end up bloated and consumed by self-loathing.

All of this take place because you haven't been listening to your body. Nobody needs to be told what foods are good for them. There can't be anybody left on the planet who thinks it's a good idea to have burger and chips for every meal. You should be eating a mix of carbohydrates, protein and fat. Don't cut one of them out because you've read a faddy diet book.

None of that is new. But for people who've spent their lives torturing themselves on strange diets, what follows might be. Eat when you're hungry. Stop when you're full. If your stomach is rumbling, or you're feeling unexpectedly weak or irritable, then they're unmistakeable signs that it's time to take more calories on. Feeling sad or lonely isn't the same trigger. Keep an eye out, watch what happens when you eat certain types of food or change your portion sizes. What gives you energy? What makes you bloated? When do you put on weight?

So, for example, the result of my observation of my appetite and the effect that food has on me is that I now only eat two main meals a day. Three, for me, is just too much, especially since the portions we consume in the West are probably equivalent to five or six meals. You just don't need that much food inside you.

But that's clearly my individual perspective, which is informed by own individual experience. It will be different for you. In fact, it *should* be different for you because your body is different and will be sending you very different messages. There's nobody better placed than you to make the right decision about what enters your mouth.

GO TO SLEEP!

Some people like to boast about going to bed at one o'clock. 'Yeah, I can live on three or four hours' sleep,' they'll say, as if it's some kind of great achievement.

I mean, of course it's *possible*, but if you have so little sleep you're making yourself more susceptible to injury and little niggles will hang around. When you haven't had enough shut-eye your brain feels as if it's fogged and hazy, and it's difficult to think and make good decisions. It can also really take a swing at your emotional resilience. You'll be snappy, you'll get burnt out.

Sleep is the process that gives our body time to perform all those vital functions that enable us to recover. While we sleep we rest, digest and repair. You might think you're being more efficient when you limit your body's ability to replenish yourself, but you'd be fooling yourself. Sleep is what gives you endurance and sustainability.

Just as with eating and exercise, take the time to find out what works for you. When I was in the Special Forces there were prolonged stretches of time during which I couldn't control when I slept and my schedule was at the mercy of the operations I was sent on. There were times when I had to go without sleep across three days and two nights. So I know at first-hand how difficult it is to recover from being deprived of sleep, and I know how emptied of energy it leaves you. That's why I'm so militant about my sleep schedule now. I've learned what works for me. I'm early to bed and early to rise.

It's largely a question of discipline. Try to go to bed at the same time each night – the more consistent you are, the better your sleep–wake cycle will work. If you want to be asleep by eleven, make sure your head is on the pillow by half-ten. Don't fuck about on your phone or watch TV. Just do it. And if you can, try to resolve any problems that are troubling you before you get into bed. (See Chapter 8 on anxiety or help on managing worries.)

I sleep well because I keep to a regular routine and I always know I've done a full day's work. I close my eyes in the knowledge that I've tried as hard as I could, given everything possible. If your body and mind aren't tired by the time you climb into bed, perhaps it's worth asking yourself if you are filling your day properly.

LESSONS

Faddy diets and get-fit-quick schemes are only ever going to be short-term fixes. But a healthy, balanced lifestyle can become the bedrock of your success.

Don't live your life on default. Make the most of every day by following a sensible routine.

Set up good habits when you're young. The older you get, the harder it becomes to change the way you eat, sleep and – most importantly – exercise.

You must constantly exercise your body *and* your mind. If you let one languish, you can be sure it will drag the other one down with it.

Your body is the best guide there is to what it needs to function at its best level. Your body is constantly communicating with you. All you have to do is listen.

Sleep isn't an optional extra. Don't make the mistake of thinking you can skip this crucial, irreplaceable chance to repair, restore and recover.

CHAPTER 5

CENTRE YOUR LIFE AROUND YOUR FAMILY

How to be a good parent.

MY CAREER AS an elite soldier meant that for many years I failed as a husband and father. It's not a nice thing to have to write, but it's true. When I was in the SBS, the military got the best parts of me. When they called, I'd come running. My family had a roof over their heads and food in their bellies, and I thought that was enough. But what they didn't have was me.

My life was military, military, military. I volunteered for everything. I volunteered for things I didn't need to do, missions that I knew could end up with my wife losing her husband and my children losing their dad. That's how committed I was. That's how little I could see how damaging my absence from family life really was. If something came up, I wouldn't waste a second thinking about anybody but myself: *I'll go in first.*

That's how, although I didn't need to do a third tour of Afghanistan with the SBS, I ended up going anyway. I'd missed the first couple of months because I was on a course. After that I was due to report for another course – I needed to revisit the qualifications I'd taken some time previously. But almost as soon as I arrived I was turning around and rushing back home – Emilie was having complications with her pregnancy. Our boy Gabriel's heartbeat was low and they'd booked her into hospital to get everything moving. This left me with a significant choice. I had a new baby to help look after and a course to finish. Because the course was overseas, I'd be able to come back every weekend. By my standards at the time, that was me being *very* present at home.

Instead I claimed that I'd an ear infection, which I knew would be enough to get me discharged from the course and sent back to Afghanistan. As I saw it, being on the frontline was my job. That was what I'd been trained to do and the reason why I'd joined the SBS. I guess I was a bit like a footballer who's been through his club's academy, who's spent years and years perfecting his talent, and is now desperate to prove how good he really is. If you're given the chance to play at the very highest level in the Champions League, are you really going to turn it down? Or are you going to ask if you can go back down to the youth teams because it's easier? Of course you're fucking not.

I was confident, I thrived on pressure and I wanted to see how good I could be. I loved the ethos and what I believed was the brotherhood. And for a while, that felt like enough for me to ignore all the signs that something wasn't quite right.

I'd go away for months at a time, leaving Emilie to cope by herself. Then I'd show up like a sudden storm, knocking to pieces the finely balanced existence Emilie had built – the existence that enabled her to cope with the unbelievable demands my career placed on her. And I was hard to deal with during those transitions, as I'd always need time to take one head off and put another on – when you've spent almost half a year kicking doors down, ordinary life is extremely difficult to adjust to. Although all around me was the clean, orderly calm of our little family home in the English countryside, when I closed my eyes I could still see the dust and squalor of Afghanistan, my nose full of the overpowering stench of aviation fuel and the grim chatter of a heavy machine gun in my ears. I wanted to be able to focus on the precious time I had with my wife and my beautiful young children, and yet I couldn't. My mind would churn away, thinking of everything I'd experienced over the last few months. I was moody, tense and easily distracted. And then by the time everything finally settled I'd be away again.

I don't think I appreciated at the time how strange and disruptive this must have been for my kids. One moment they were living a normal existence, the next this bearded, battle-scarred stranger was walking through the door. I remember coming back after one tour to find that our daughter Shyla, who was one at the time, barely recognised me. It still hurts me to this day to think of the look on her face as she pushed me away when I tried to hold her. I carried on talking to her, thinking that I could find a way of making her see who I was and how much I loved her. But nothing I could say worked. She stared at me blankly. To her I was no more significant than the guy who'd been round earlier that week to fix the boiler. And although I knew I couldn't show her how cut up I was, inside I was dying. I didn't give up. I couldn't give up.

A couple of days later, Emilie came in and found me sitting on the floor playing with Barbies, doing everything I could to get even a tiny smile from my daughter. She thought I'd lost the plot. All Emilie had seen since I'd been back had been a pent-up war machine, and now here I was doing silly voices and waving dolls around. Almost the worst thing was that it was just at the moment that Shyla had finally come to accept me again that I had to put my uniform back on and head back to Afghanistan.

What breaks my heart is that it took me so long for me to realise how wrong I'd got everything. In fact the penny didn't drop until well after I had left the military. I had to be thrown into fucking *prison* before I actually understood how far short I'd fallen. By then I wasn't even doing the bare minimum like I'd done before. You can't provide for your family when you're behind bars and you certainly can't be there for your kids when they need you most.

It was in jail that I saw Emilie was there for me when I'd been abandoned by almost everybody from my life in uniform. But then she'd always been there for me – there had never been a second when she had not been supporting me, or sacrificing herself. It's just that I was so blinded by my devotion to my career that I could not see it. She understood I'd given everything I could to the armed forces. I thought that my devotion would be returned, but instead I came to realise that they saw me as a highly trained but replaceable piece of meat.

I'm trying to do everything I can to make amends, although I'm not sure if I'll ever be able to quite make up for my absences and failures. It still eats me up. I'm not here to give myself excuses. I was selfish – my shortcomings as a father were mine, nobody else's. But I think maybe I'd have found it easier to get my priorities in line if my own father hadn't died when I was so young. His death deprived me of that positive role model we all need. It's all very well reading about what it means to be a good parent. You have to *see* it with your own eyes too.

Instead I had to figure it out as I went along. I started out as a dad without any clear idea of how it should be done. I chose the easy route – joining the army, getting married early, taking up the option of having a military house. I did all the things that I thought were expected of me. You could say I was living on default, never really interrogating the situation to ask myself whether it really was the best thing for me and my family.

These days I'm most at peace once I'm back at home. I think it's because my focus isn't on myself, it's on my children. I'm there every day, buzzing around with the attention span of a gnat. I love being a father. I love being a provider. I love going out there and working fucking hard. Love it. Because I can go back and share the rewards with my family and everyone else I care for.

I now see work as the thing that supports my family, not the other way round. That doesn't mean I'm not passionate about everything I do, but it does mean my priorities have shifted. Every job, every business relationship, will come to an end some day. Your family will always be there. If I fail at work I can always find another project. If my family falls apart then I'll be spending the rest of my life trying to pick up the pieces. I see my family as being an ecosystem. What happens inside that ecosystem is what really matters. Nothing else has the same value.

Most of all, I now know this – being a father isn't something you can half-do. It's not something you can be a success at if you're only using the dregs left over from the other parts of your life. You're not just a father at the weekends, or in the holidays, or in the gaps between seeing your mates, or when you're feeling well rested, or when there's no other option. You're a father every single second of the day. You're a father even when you're ill, or knackered, or would prefer to be doing literally anything other than wiping a child's bottom. You have to give the best of yourself to this insane, demanding, magical project. As I see it, there's no part of my existence in which the stakes are higher, or the rewards greater.

THE RESPONSIBILITY THAT NEVER ENDS

People prioritise work and they don't even realise it. They will bend over backwards to support their team at work, and then they're so lazy at home that they expect their family to do everything for them.

You get men who stride into the kitchen after they've finished work thinking their day is done. They're just there, asking 'Where's my dinner?' and telling their kids to shut up so that they can 'finally get some peace'. I fucking *hate* that. I don't want to be one of those people who can't wait to get back to the office. What kind of an existence is that? I'm never in a million years going to be just sitting there yelling for them to bring me a can of beer. I couldn't live with myself if I became that man.

I'm as professional at home as I am at work. Probably more so. Of course I'm not perfect. Just as I don't always get things right in my career, I don't always get things right when I'm around my family. But that's not for lack of effort. It's too easy to get complacent. You wouldn't rest on your laurels at work, so why do you think you can do the same when it comes to your marriage or your children?

The second I walk through my front door I know that I've instantly got a hundred times more responsibility than I do when I'm working. If I'm lounging on the couch during the day and my kids are up and about, then I'm doing something wrong. I want to be on it all the time. There will be plenty of opportunities for relaxation once they're in bed.

Remember this: your children didn't ask to be born. They don't exist to fill some gaping emotional hole inside you. They don't owe you anything. They are your responsibility. And it's a responsibility that doesn't end when they turn eighteen or get married or have kids. It's up to you to make sure that your children get the best possible start. But it's also a lifelong project. I'll be there for my kids until I take my last breath.

As parents it will be you who plays a central part in shaping your children's minds. I think teachers are so important, but their responsibility starts and finishes in the classroom. They can teach my kids about maths, history and good grammar. Everything else is up to us as parents. Our job is to teach them about *life*.

Everyone will have a view on how that can be achieved. I respect everyone else's opinion. Mine is based on what I've experienced myself – of my dad dying when I was young. His death created a hole in my life that I don't know if I'll ever fill. Having a positive father figure is something I believe is really important.

I've seen what they can learn from me, and what they can learn from Emilie. We can teach them a great deal, but I'm also adamant that they must learn to think for themselves, which is harder than it might seem, because they spend so much of their time in institutions that are dedicated to trying to control their every move.

I make sure my children are self-sufficient. I want them to do chores. There are six of us in the house. Everyone has to pull their weight. We don't really need their help to keep everything going, and yet by contributing they're finding out what it means to be given responsibility. These are jobs that aren't beyond them, stuff that any kid their age could do. Small stuff. But it will all help them learn what work means, that life isn't just handed to you on a plate.

It's all preparation for the big wide world that one day they're going to be stepping out into.

BUILD THE WALL

Some people think there's something glamorous about spinning plates, that people who make work calls while they're knocking up their kids' dinners are somehow heroic, that it's fine for your mind to be in two places at once. That's utter bollocks. You have to build a wall between your professional and personal lives. At work you should be thinking 100 per cent about your job. At home you should be thinking 100 per cent about your family. I do my work as quickly and efficiently as possible so that I can come home and know that everything else is squared away. I won't let myself sit at the dinner table thinking about this or that job. That was true to some extent when I was in the Special Forces, but it's certainly the case now. Your kids will notice if you're preoccupied, and you're going to be a far less effective parent if half your brain is taken up with thoughts about work.

But more than that, I believe it's your responsibility to shield your children from the stresses and strains of adult life. They don't need to hear you complaining about how your manager is giving you a hard time at work. They shouldn't be exposed to your money worries. That's your business, not theirs. You can't heap adult concerns onto their young shoulders. Let your children enjoy their childhood.

I'm always telling my own kids, 'Don't think you need to grow up too quick.' When you're eighteen, you'll be an adult. If you live to be a hundred, you'll have had eighty-two years of being an adult. Don't make that stressful and demanding portion of your time on this planet any longer than it needs to be. You've got *plenty* of time to be a grown-up; plenty of time to wish that you were still young and carefree and untroubled by all the complexities that come with growing older. I want to preserve their innocence for as long as possible.

This isn't the same as wrapping them up in cotton wool. Elsewhere in this book I'll talk about how important it is to challenge your kids. I don't want them growing up thinking they're little princes and princesses who never need to lift a finger. They've got to be resilient and resourceful, with the ability to solve problems by themselves – even if they know that I will *always*, under *any* circumstances, be there for them if they need me.

LEADERS OF THE PACK

You and your partner are leaders of a pack. The family is the ultimate team. If you don't stimulate, challenge and work on and with each other then of course it will go stale. It might even break up.

As leaders of the pack, you're the ones who are responsible for the mood in your home. That mood is very often dictated by the nature of your relationship with your partner. I understand that the state of my bond with Emilie is crucial to the well-being of everyone else under our roof. If we're at each other's throats it's going to have a massive knock-on effect on our children. You should always be conscious of the energy you emit and the impact it will have on anybody who comes into contact with you.

As I've said before, children don't listen to much you tell them, but they're watching *everything* you do. They're scrutinising you without you even realising. That's how they learn about the world and how to exist within it. Every time you walk into the same room as them, you're teaching them a lesson. What do you want them to see?

What sort of energy are you emitting? If you're feeling shit, be open about it. Tell them what's wrong and why. Your kids aren't dumb, you can't fool them. Don't snap at them, or mumble under your breath and claim that nothing is up. All you'll achieve is convincing everyone in a 100-metre radius that you're a miserable cunt.

You're only human, so of course you'll have arguments with your partner. But next time it's got to the stage where you're tempted to start screaming obscenities, remember who might be listening and what effect it might have on them. What kind of lesson will it teach them? How will it make them feel to see their parents behaving aggressively? It's a million times better to resolve your disagreements in a positive and respectful fashion. If you're feeling angry or upset, don't sulk and create bad vibes that will seep into every corner of the house. Get over yourself!

If I feel that Emilie is exuding negativity I'll tell her straight away. 'If I can feel it, the kids are going to feel it. Let's flip that into a positive.' And she'll say exactly the same to me. I think it's really important to try to balance out the energy in the house. I can't be doing with the sort of atmosphere where the room is full of tension or unresolved grievances. It sends me off my head, it's my kryptonite. I can't settle until it's sorted out. To avoid it, I act as a mediator. If any of my kids have had a fight, I'll make sure they apologise to each other and clear the air.

I'm so adamant about this that I think they must sometimes get sick of me. I'm always there asking, 'Why are you negative? Why are you miserable?'

Last of all, always remember that you have to protect your family. You can't allow a bad atmosphere to creep in. If someone else outside of your family is behaving in a way that negatively colours the mood in any way, then you must act. (For the best ways to conduct difficult conversations, see Chapter 14 on the power of saying No.)

HAPPY FAMILIES ARE NO ACCIDENT

I'm not naïve. I know that time and circumstance can prevent you from being the parent you want to be. But I don't understand those fathers and mothers who are fatalistic about their families – the type that think that it's just a matter of chance that some families get on and others don't, or that some kids remember to say please and thank you, while others zoom out of the room without so much as a second glance.

Instead of working at the problem and trying to solve what's wrong, they just shrug their shoulders and pour themselves another glass of rosé. I pay attention to my family. I apply myself to identifying what their problems are. I make it my business to know what's going on with them. That's because I want to do everything I can to help them all thrive.

The thing is, children don't need much. They need to feel secure, they need to feel loved and they want a bit of guidance. When children misbehave, the majority of the time it's because they want some form of attention.

That's why Emilie and I put a lot of effort in to building a home environment that's fun and honest, and full of enough activity to stimulate both body and mind. We work our arses off to pass on the values and attitudes that we believe are important. I'm not going to lie, it would be far easier to stick our kids in front of an iPad or blame somebody else when they act up. But the net result of the work we've invested in is that my children are polite, respectful and honest, and they can engage in a conversation (all things that to me are far more important than whether or not they're smashing it at school).

This is the product of the discipline and structure that we've introduced into our home. I'm not talking about being a drill sergeant. I don't shout or scream or impose arbitrary rules. As I understand it, discipline is actually about organisation. It's preparing my kids' packed lunches the night before so that we don't wake up in a rush the next morning. It's making sure they go to bed early enough to get a proper sleep. All of this requires constant effort. It demands being alert to their changing needs. But it's worth it.

The effect on a child's mental well-being of the absence of discipline and structure goes way beyond whatever minor trouble you experience because none of you had your shit together enough to get them on the school bus on time. Missing a bus once is a short-term inconvenience. Waking up in a negative environment day after day after fucking day is a long-term catastrophe.

Of course, discipline and structure aren't the same as being rigid and stuck in your ways. You have to leave space for spontaneity. And I also know that you cannot operate at full tilt twenty-four hours a day, 365 days a year. Although we don't want our children to make a habit of sitting down with an iPad and ignoring the rest of the world or locking themselves in their rooms, there will always be days when Gabriel will want to play on his Xbox from breakfast to dinner – and I'll let him. Remember that kids are kids. If you wake up and they just want to laze around on the couch for a while, that's fine. Join them! It's good to break things up from time to time. I've found that the fact that I have to travel so often for work has helped strengthen our family. It gives us natural breaks. I might hate the fact that I'm on the other side of the world and can't give Emilie and the kids a cuddle. But it also means we aren't always under each other's feet.

ONE OTHER THING to remember is that being firm isn't the same as being aggressive. You can change the tone of your voice if they're cheeky with their mum or refusing to go to bed, but I'm 100 per cent never physical with my children. I don't believe in smacking them. I'm never going to say to them, 'Fucking tell me or I'll whack you.' You can scare your kids into saying or doing whatever you want. But that doesn't mean that you should.

What I will do is sit them down and talk about the consequences of their actions, for them and for others. Kids need to understand the effect of what they do or say has on the people around them. They need to be aware of the situation they're in, and what the appropriate responses to it might be.

Before I say anything else I tell them that I love and care for them. It creates the context for everything that follows, because they know that I'm not doing this just for the hell of it or because I want to get one-up on a thirteen-year-old. As a result, my kids feel that they can come to me when they've fucked up. They know I'm not going to scream and shout at them. They also know that I'll treat them with respect, and explain what I'm doing and why. The chances are they won't like my reasons, but at least they'll know what they are. If I've got to tell them that they can't have a sleepover, I'll remind them that it's because they were away the previous weekend. Or if I stop them from going out into the woods late in the evening, I'll explain why it might be dangerous to do so.

There are lots of occasions in my life when the chief instructor has an important role to play. My relationship with my kids is definitely not one of them.

THE SACRIFICE QUESTION

What are you willing to sacrifice to be the best parent that you can be? You can't have it all. You can't give 100 per cent to everything. That's just a fact. It's also something that means you have to make difficult choices. You can't pretend that you're the same person with the same life as you were before having kids. Something has to give. It might be nights out with your mates, it might be the leisurely round of golf you play every Sunday, it might be the season ticket to the club you support. If you can't put your child's needs ahead of your own, then why would you even bring them into the world at all?

LESSONS

Being a parent isn't a part-time job. It's the most important role you'll ever play – more than your job, more than anything. You have to give your children the best of you.

Your children didn't ask to be born. You have a responsibility to them and their welfare that will not end until the day you take your last breath.

Putting food on the table is just a start. A parent is more than a provider.

Don't force your kids to deal with your problems. Your children don't need to know about your troubles with your boss, or that tricky situation you're in with a client. When you walk through that door, you're a parent, not an employee. Act like it.

Set the right example. Your children might not *listen* to a word you say, but you better fucking believe that they'll see and hear everything that goes on under your roof. So if you can't tell them how to become a good human being, then make sure that you show them by setting the right example.

Families don't fix themselves. You can't sit back and hope that your children will muddle along. Make it your business to find out their problems. Give them the discipline and structure they need to thrive.

CHAPTER 6

EMBRACE FAILURE

Turn setbacks into opportunities and make failure the engine for your success.

LET'S BE HONEST. If you're in the public eye and you've been cancelled, you've certainly experienced a setback. It's the most public kind of failure. Some people don't survive the pressure that follows: the media free-for-all, the speculation, the constant attacks on your character, the hurt that it causes your family.

Many people reading this will already know, or think they know, the story of how my time with the UK version of *SAS: Who Dares Wins* came to an end. It was in all the papers, after all – every one of them from the *Sun* to the *Guardian*. So there's nothing more to say … except, of course, that the story is more complicated than you might imagine.

What you should know is that well before they announced that I was going to be axed from the show, the production company knew that I wanted to leave. It had been on the cards for ages. I'd been enduring rather than enjoying it for a while and, in fact, I'd had to be talked into doing the last series by my management team. I already felt that the show had become too scripted, and that health and safety had become too powerful. It had drifted away from what had made it so fun and exciting to be a part of.

It felt as if rather than being there to facilitate things, health and safety were actually calling the shots. I wasn't being allowed to do my work in the way that I wanted it to be done, which, let's remember, was a big reason behind why the show was so successful in the first place. I thought we'd come to the end of the road and it would be best for everyone if we could part ways in a healthy, positive way. Making that show was for a long time an amazing experience for me, and it undeniably changed my life. I'd made great friends, met some unbelievable inspiring people and didn't want to do anything that would sour those memories.

But against my better instincts I got talked into going back up to Scotland to film another series. This time round, I quickly discovered that the health and safety stuff that had bugged me so much in the previous series had got even worse. In the past, they'd sign off an entire area. Once they said we were good to go, we had free rein. But now health and safety was being addressed on a task-by-task basis. There was no longer any room for spontaneity, for the sorts of challenges that really tested the contestants.

My frustrations came to a head when we did the fast-rope pick-up, where contestants who have been treading water then get hauled up onto a moving boat by their partners. Everything had started OK. They all swam out, did what they needed to do with varying degrees of success, and they came back to the shore, where, still dripping wet, I made them sit on their Bergens. I wanted to condition them to the elements. The more they got accustomed to being soaking cold now, the easier it would become as the course progressed – their discomfort would stop being a distraction.

They were all shivering, looking at me for their next instruction. 'We're going back in that water,' I shouted. 'You think this is over. It's not. Ignore the elements!'

Just as I was walking them back I could hear a commotion behind me. I briefly thought, *What the hell's going on?* but before I could even try to find out, some of the contestants had already started splashing into the water. Once everyone was in far enough that the water reached their chests, I got them to bend their heads down so that they were just submerged.

All of a sudden one of the commissioners came up to me and said, 'Ant! Red flag! Red flag! Red flag! You need to get them out of the water!'

Shit, I thought, *something dramatic must have happened somewhere else.* Red flags were only called when there had been a real breach of the health and safety rules, the kind that involved a serious injury, or even a death. I felt a surge of adrenaline, and desperately hoped that everybody was OK. I knew that everything in front of me was fine, but what about elsewhere? All of the worst-possible scenarios played through my head. Had one of the safety boats turned over?

So I brought the bewildered recruits back, then headed over to the production office to ask them what the Code Red was for.

'Well, Ant, it was you.'

'We were fucking fine! There was nothing wrong with us.'

'You put them back in the water after the task. Why did you do that?'

'What do you mean?'

'You put them in above waist height.'

'They'd just been treading water as part of the exercises,' I explained, 'and they were already as wet as they could possibly get. Are you fucking kidding me? You called Code Red because of *that*?'

The whole thing was an exercise in ticking boxes. It was like a decision had been made to put health and safety in charge of the whole show, while I was just there to decorate proceedings by yelling at the appropriate points. Fuck. That.

I then lost it. 'Unless this changes,' I shouted, 'I'm fucking leaving. I'll walk off set. I cannot have my recruits interrupted halfway through a task. You're going to ruin the whole authenticity of the show. It's out of hand!'

Things didn't get any better, and there followed flashpoint after flashpoint, with every task seeming to be interrupted for any number of bullshit reasons. On other occasions I felt like the production company were pursuing agendas that really affected the integrity of the show. Stuff happened that I just couldn't believe.

Again and again I threatened to walk off, and I was probably yelling at the production team more than I was at the recruits. I was always willing to butt heads if I thought that the authenticity of the show was being further eroded or if some other element of what we were doing was being compromised.

Ultimately, however, I still had a job to do. So did everybody else. As miserable as it was making us, we completed the show. But that was it for me. As soon as I was back I let my agency know that I wanted out. I even said as much to one of the producers. 'You guys are going to be getting a call very soon,' I told him. 'I don't agree with the way the course is being run. I'm not being allowed to do my job anymore. I'm out.'

What happened next was a bit strange. My agency tried to set up a call with the production company. Every time a conversation was arranged, it got put off. Something was up, but we weren't sure what. After six weeks of this madness, the call finally took place. People had barely finished saying their hellos when Minnow announced that having spoken to Channel 4 they'd decided that they wouldn't be working with me anymore.

Within forty minutes of the call ending, the *Mirror*, the *Sun* and the *Daily Mail* had run pieces announcing that I'd been sacked. My production company had read the runes, and I'd given them plenty of warning. They knew that I was going to jump so they pushed me first. And to be honest, I don't even blame them. They were just doing what they thought they needed to do – protecting their brand – although precisely what that brand is now, I'm not too sure. The first series of the show was so exciting and so real because of its brutality. We weren't pretending to be anything other than what we were: uncompromising alpha males from the military. That's obviously the opposite of the show that Channel 4 and Minnow want now. The woke patrol have got their victory, and I'll be very interested to see where the series goes next.

But I'm not going to bother rehearsing the reckless, desperate allegations and statements that were made about me. It's boring, pointless and won't achieve anything. I've got nothing to hide or feel ashamed of. I'm as happy now as I was then to air anything they think needs to be aired in court. Of course, that's not going to happen. It was all just smoke and mirrors. All I will say is, if you never want to work with me again, if my behaviour and views are genuinely so out of step with your channel's values, then fine, I can live with that. But don't say that and then have me on-screen a few months later in a different show. That just doesn't stack up.

I'll hold my hands up to the stuff I know I did wrong. I clearly wasn't an easy person to work with on that last series. I was so angry and frustrated for so much of it that I did behave in a way I'm not proud of. I never thought I'd be the guy threatening to walk off set. Sure, I can point to reasons why I did lose my rag, but the point is, I shouldn't have let myself go. There's a chapter in this book on controlling your emotions. There's another on how to have productive confrontations. I didn't do either. In the process, I failed to live up to the standards I set myself. I regret that. I really fucking regret that.

The whole affair was a setback for me, and I hated being part of a media storm. More than that, I hated the impact that all the innuendo and gossip about me had on my family. It wasn't just the fallout from my 'sacking', and the hits I've taken to my own reputation and my relationships with companies; it was also the whole experience of filming a series I hadn't even wanted to be part of.

And yet it's also been a clean break that has liberated me. The show was dragging me down and had got to the point where I felt as if each time I went to do another series I was taking a step back rather than a step forward.

I've learned lessons and I've grown more resilient. It taught me a lot about people's real priorities. I understand now that there's no loyalty in TV. Channels and production companies are too interested in jumping on fads. What's the next clickbait? What's going to grab attention? People don't mean much to them. It's all business. It's all money.

Some brands and charities I thought I had strong connections with announced that they didn't want to be associated with me anymore. That hurt, but it certainly clarified a few things. All the cobwebs have been cleared out and my life is now far more free from hangers-on than it was before.

I DON'T TAKE LOSSES,
I TAKE LESSONS

I failed twice to make it into P Company; I quit the army before I ever got going; my first marriage fell apart; I was thrown out of the Metropolitan Police; I've been banned for drink-driving; I spent time in prison; my contract for the UK version of *SAS: Who Dares Wins* was not renewed; for years I failed to be the father I should have been; I didn't make it to the summits of the Matterhorn, Aconcagua and Elbrus.

I've listed these – a small and far from exhaustive selection of my failures – because I'm not ashamed of any of them. You should never feel embarrassed to have failed. It's part of life, like breathing. I've had a million times more failures than successes. Every day the total of my failures increases, and that's going to continue until I take my last breath.

But I wouldn't change any of them, because each one has played its part in making me the human being I am now. Failure has assumed such a huge role in my life that I've come to see it as a positive force. Embrace it, learn how to use it to your advantage.

Failure builds resilience. It pushes your brain into overload. And it's the best education there is, as nothing helps you grow like being knocked down. You don't learn anything when you win but you get handed a whole fucking lot of lessons when you lose. It's the most intense, most thrilling, most productive way of learning that I know. And there's nothing academic or theoretical about the lessons it teaches you. They're rooted in real-life experience.

Society, however, has made people scared of failure. It has made 'failure' a dirty word and is trying to create a world in which nobody can ever fail. It sometimes seems that society doesn't want us to realise what we're capable of; it doesn't want us to push past our limits and beyond.

This is why I'm so against school sports days where there aren't firsts, seconds, thirds and fourths. Where there aren't winners and losers, and everybody gets a fucking badge at the end of the day. It's dehumanising. I genuinely think it's taking a big chunk out of what it means to be a human being. It's as if we're determined to put evolution into reverse. If you aren't willing to commit to something where failure is a very real possibility then ultimately you're neglecting yourself. You're ensuring that you'll miss out on all those opportunities to grow and learn. You're ensuring that part of who you are and what you're capable of will be hidden forever. Talent without hard work is just talent. Nothing more. If you're not willing to expose yourself to failure, if you're not willing to put that graft in, get better at it, learn from your mistakes, what you've got will always remain potential. And potential never got anybody anywhere.

The people who open themselves up to failure, who know that they're going to fail more often than succeed and have made their peace with that idea – they're the ones who are going to figure life out more quickly. Make sure you're one of them.

DON'T BE AFRAID OF FAILURE

If you don't make mistakes in life, you don't make anything. Failure is the precondition for success. You have to commit to it. Once you've done that, everything will fall into place.

If you look at the world honestly you'll see that failure is all around us. So it makes sense to try to turn it to our benefit rather than letting it crush us. Often the reason we don't is because we can't see past the short-term pain involved. People think – usually quite wrongly – that this timid mindset is the safest place to be.

People fail once and it changes their whole attitude towards the world. Something will happen and they'll say to themselves, 'Well, I'm not going to go near *that* again.' And our lives revolve around those decisions we do and don't take. An entire existence can be altered by something that occurs in our brains for five or ten seconds. 'I wish I'd done that' or 'I wish I'd done this'. I know loads of ex-military guys who are going to spend the rest of their time on this planet saying to anybody who'll listen, 'I wish I'd gone on Selection.' Well, why didn't you? Mostly they'll say something like, 'Oh, it wasn't the right time.' The more honest ones will be more straight: 'I was afraid of failing.'

People are afraid of failure, but why? If I'd gone on Selection and failed, I'd have been disappointed – it's always hard to put so much effort into something that doesn't work out. There would have been a blow to my ego and I'd guess that there would have been a bit of banter from some of the lads whom I'd told I was giving it a go. But otherwise? Probably nothing. The chances are I'd have had another go the next time I was able to. In our heads we build failure up to be some sort of massive catastrophe. And yet in truth most failures pass unnoticed by the world at large. Failures are generally only as big as we make them.

When you learn to embrace failure, you're taking the first step on the way to avoiding being the sort of bitter creature who slumps in the corner of a pub, making a whole pint last an evening, saying over and over again to nobody in particular, 'I wish I'd tried …'

I go through life not giving a fuck about whether I fail. That's why my career is so varied. I've tried a million things because I'm not afraid of getting stuff wrong. There's no reason why everybody can't do the same.

One thing you need to understand is that you can't lead a risk-free life. The second you get into a car or step onto a bus or a plane, you're taking a risk. But you've already calculated that the upside of being able to visit your mates or go on holiday is worth that small risk. It's a risk stepping outside your front door! It's a risk never stepping outside your front door!

You can reframe your thinking. You can either say I took a risk by putting myself forward for Selection, or you could say that the bigger risk was to *not* try. Passing Selection opened my life up completely. Being in the SBS was one of the most rewarding, exhilarating experiences a human being can have. The same is true of agreeing to go on *SAS: Who Dares Wins*. Clearly there were risks. I had a growing security business, the Special Forces hierarchy were firmly against it, and if it had gone tits up I might have opened myself up to ridicule. And yet look at the upside. If you focus too much on what might happen if things go badly, you might lose sight of all the good things that could come your way if things go well.

How are you going to find your passion in life if you spend your entire time worrying about getting your fingers burned?

So I invest my money because I know that it could potentially give me a much greater return than leaving it mouldering in the bank. I put some aside for a rainy day, sure, but the rest I try to make work for me. I know that some investments will pay off, and some won't. That's a risk I'm willing to take. I'd far rather get out there and try rather than being one of those people who is always waiting for the 'right moment'.

THE PAST IS JUST DATA

If you've had a disappointment, it's OK to have a sulk. Pretending you're happy isn't healthy. But as you sit there in the aftermath of a failure, surveying the ruins and the debris, it's important to keep a healthy sense of perspective.

It doesn't matter if you've crashed and burned. You're still fucking here. The world hasn't ended. You're still fucking breathing, you're still fucking fighting. And you're in good company. The stories of the greatest men and women in history are littered with examples of failures they experienced. And guess what? They always managed to pick themselves up and go again. You can do the same thing.

Make sure you don't fall into the trap of being one of those people who fail once and immediately decide that they're a failure, with that idea overwhelming their whole identity and paralysing them. You shouldn't let yourself be defined by your failures, just as you shouldn't be defined by your successes.

What's happened to you is just an event in a lifetime full of them. It would be ridiculous to call Muhammad Ali a failure because he lost a few bouts. And nobody's ever going to accuse Leonardo da Vinci of being a washout because some of his inventions didn't end up panning out.

Personally, I never dwell on the past. I've never wanted to be one of those people who do one decent thing and then spend the next twenty years milking the shit out of it. For me there's no difference between my many failures and my far fewer successes. There's no hierarchy – they all have the same value. They're all part of the roadmap that has made me who I am today. They're all just moments in time. I don't want to be known for something I once did, whether it was good or bad. I don't want anything in my past to limit me or exclusively define who I am. When something is behind me and I've drawn all the lessons I can from the experience, I don't have much use for it. It's done and dusted. The past is just data.

Mourn the failure, extract everything positive you can from it, then move on. Don't waste time wallowing. Don't pretend you can turn the clock back to a time before everything went wrong. Instead, start planning what you're going to do next. If you've had to pull out of a marathon because you picked up an injury, start thinking about what marathon you can enter as soon as you're recovered. If you've failed your driving test, book another!

The longer you wait, the more difficult it will be to establish the momentum you need to go out there again. It's amid the wreckage caused by your failure that you can start building the foundations of your next success.

IT'S NOT PERSONAL

In my experience of talking to other soldiers, a lot of their post-traumatic stress disorder comes from them taking situations personally. They jump through a door with their mate, and their mate gets taken out by the Taliban who was waiting for them. Now, the Taliban doesn't care know or care who you are. He's just there to defend his boss. If someone comes through that door, they're going to get sprayed. But the guy who makes it out of there personalises the situation: why wasn't it me? I should have taken that bullet.

It was never personal for me. I went into every combat situation with the same mindset: I've got a job to do. It didn't matter if the Taliban commander we were after was responsible for IEDs that had killed twenty Marines or if he was telling kids to push wheelbarrows full of explosives into the path of British patrols and detonating them from a safe distance.

That attitude has helped me avoid making failure personal. This is a really important principle to bear in mind. Don't fall into the trap of thinking that your setbacks are the result of you being a bad person, or that you somehow deserved to fail. There will be times when you don't get a job because the company who advertised the role had a very narrow conception of the sort of person whom they wanted to fill it. If you don't get the job because you pissed around and didn't prepare, then that's on you. You fucking should take responsibility for that. But if the reason you weren't offered the job is because the firm had already decided who they wanted to hire, then you cannot possibly see that as a failure. The world moves along very straight lines these days. People like to put other people in very specific boxes. It's more important to stay true to your beliefs than it is to mould yourself in a doomed attempt to please others.

When something bad happens to you, don't make a hard situation worse than it needs to be by blaming yourself. Most relationships end because the two people involved have drifted apart. If that's the case, then why make an unpleasant moment in your life even worse by sinking into a pit of self-recrimination: 'There must be something wrong with me'; 'Oh, if only I'd said or done this, it could have been different'; 'It's all my fault'. And whatever you do, don't start catastrophising – 'I'm never going to get another girlfriend!' – because whatever is going on inside your head becomes your reality. If you create a nightmare, you're most probably going to have to live in it.

TAKE YOUR TIME

One of the problems we have nowadays is that we're in an era where people expect immediate success. People are too quick to say, 'Oh, I tried that and didn't get anywhere. I think it's time to bin it off.' But it just doesn't work like that. How do you know that your lucky break isn't five years down the line? You don't build a career in five minutes. Most of the time it takes years. My books, my tours, my TV shows – none of that happened overnight. They're the product of everything I've done and learned and fucked up at since I was a kid.

So, if you've had a setback, remind yourself that this is just one small moment in what will probably be a really successful life. You may even look back on it as the start of something, not the end.

I've started and stopped right throughout my life. I've tried and failed. Some things I've loved and stuck at for years. Some things were good for a while, but eventually it was time to move on. Others simply didn't work out at all. I'm sure I'll change again. I loved my time as a soldier, and I've loved my time as a TV presenter and author. But those things won't last forever. Maybe I'll get into business or fashion or film. Who knows?

What I am sure of, though, is that there's no need to rush the process. You hear people say in a pompous voice: 'The one thing we don't have is time.' I think: *Fucking hell, time is the one thing we* do *have.* Don't think you've got to settle before it gets too late. And don't ever think that that one setback means that it's time to shelve any of your dreams or ambitions. Be patient.

ONE LINK IN A CHAIN

We tend to think of failures as isolated events that go nowhere, as the disappointing end to an otherwise promising journey. I think that's a really negative way of approaching the subject.

If you look beyond the stories of mankind's greatest achievements, you'll see that very often they're building on a foundation of failures. Think of the moon landings, among the most exciting, amazing things we have achieved as a species.

Each failure the Apollo programme experienced on the way to that amazing day when Neil Armstrong took his giant leap for mankind, whether it was the Apollo 1 fire or Armstrong's close escape in the Lunar Landing Research Vehicle, brought them closer to their goal. These failures weren't cul de sacs, simply rungs on a ladder. Each time the scientists and astronauts on the programme learned a little more, gained a bit more experience.

I'm not afraid to fail ten times on my way to a single success. You can pretend that nobody's watching, but I prefer to see failure as an exercise in problem-solving. You haven't quite got it right this time, indeed you might still fall short next time. But every attempt pushes you a little further forward.

IT'S ON YOU

When you've suffered a setback, it's essential that you take full responsibility for what happened and why. The buck stops with you. The very worst thing that you can do is blame other people or bad luck, or complain about your circumstances.

If you blame other people, if you don't take responsibility, you're denying yourself the opportunity to learn something from that failure. This is the time when you have to really work. I break every setback down, analyse it, then move forward. It forces me to see where I'm vulnerable, where my weaknesses lie. Nobody is ever going to become the best versions of themselves if they don't open themselves up to failure and everything that follows from it.

So when you do experience failure, work hard to draw every lesson you can from it. As always, you've got to be brutally honest. What went wrong? Why did it go wrong? What could you have done better? Rip yourself to shreds. If you pull your punches or tell yourself a nice fairy tale about what happened, you won't be doing yourself any favours. Whatever momentary comfort you gain will be massively outweighed by the loss of a valuable chance to learn and grow.

I was one of the many people who learned some difficult lessons during the pandemic. If I say that there were two posts I put up on social media that got me into trouble over the course of 2020, you'll probably know exactly what I mean. You might agree with what I said, you might not. But I do regret posting them. Clearly, I could have worded them better. The points I wanted to make got taken out of context and I caused upset, which was never my intention.

I could have blamed other people for exaggerating or misinterpreting what I said, but that at best would have only been half the story. At the end of the day, only one person put those posts together, and only one person pressed send: me. If you blame other people for mistakes you've made, you won't solve the problem; you're just going to ensure you make the same mistakes, over and over again.

The incidents made me realise that if I'm someone who claims to be preaching positivity, venting like that doesn't have any place in my life. If I'm frustrated about something, it's far better and more constructive to go for a run than write a couple hastily conceived social media posts. What did I really think I would achieve? That I'd be able to enter into a constructive dialogue with people? The *best* I could hope for was getting something off my chest. As it was, I managed to cause a media shitshow. Those posts took maybe thirty seconds each to compose but led to months of hassle, so they're something I steer clear of now. Everything I do has to be progressive. It's got to be the beginning of a positive conversation. If it's defensive, I won't voice it.

The success of the Italian and English football teams at Euro 2020 was built on past failures. Both sides had experienced traumatic disappointments over the last five years, yet to their great credit they sat down, looked at what they'd been doing wrong and initiated huge structural changes. They realised that they'd been left behind by modern football. In response they brought in new cultures, new systems, even new ways of playing. And the net result was the complete revitalisation of their fortunes. But none of that would have happened if they hadn't failed and then been willing to learn lessons from that failure.

Although you have to be unsparing when you search for what went wrong, it's important to remember to devote time to drawing out what positives you can from the situation. Celebrate what went well. Try to make a note of any new information you gathered.

I didn't reach the summits of the Matterhorn, Aconcagua and Elbrus. In that sense, each of these attempts might be considered a failure. And yet I gained confidence, because I demonstrated to myself that I could make significant progress up a big mountain. The harsh conditions I met on each of these peaks prepared me for the epic snowstorm that would later envelop me on Mount Everest. Even during the course of the attempts I picked up so much that improved me as a climber.

So although technically speaking they were failures, I look back on them as being really positive experiences. I wouldn't have been able to reach the top of the world without them.

FAILURE IS THE ENGINE FOR GROWTH

Failure gives you the opportunity to re-evaluate yourself. If you're *not* failing, if there isn't occasionally friction between you and the world you interact with, then you probably have been sliding through life on autopilot, taking the easy route.

You'll be saying things because you know they grease the wheels, not because they're a true reflection of you and how you feel. You're doing the same things over and over again, trapped in a comfortable routine that never stretches you and never allows you to grow or learn. When you find yourself thinking that because things are ticking along OK, there's no need to ever change, then you're actually in a really dangerous place.

Sometimes things have run their course. Sometimes things need to come to an end. Sometimes what looks like failure is actually the best thing that could happen to you.

So although when it all comes crashing down it seems like a disaster, it can also end up becoming an amazing opportunity. Leaving *SAS: Who Dares Wins* has liberated me. It has given me the freedom to start again, to try new things. The break-up of my first marriage is another example. On the outside the failure of a relationship looks pretty bad, and it's the kind of thing that can end up sitting heavily on someone's shoulders. But it was clear that although day-to-day things were OK, neither of us were happy. Our marriage was going nowhere. If we'd stayed together we'd have just spent the rest of our lives making each other miserable.

'FUCK YOU' IS AN AMAZING FUEL

Don't let anything I've said so far fool you. Although I believe with every fibre of my being that you can turn failure into a positive experience, that doesn't mean that at the time it occurs failure feels anything but very fucking negative. Losing, falling short, getting things wrong: all of these hurt. In fact they can be devastating.

I see that as all the more reason to try to turn a horrendous moment into a positive. Say you've failed at something publicly, there are people laughing at you, and you feel wounded and humiliated. What better motivation can you have to help pick yourself up and get going again than the idea of proving all the doubters wrong? Use the memory to push you to try harder, to get you through moments when you might feel tempted to slacken or give up – surely anything is better than feeling that way again.

If I'm playing basketball with my twelve-year-old I'll whip his ass. I'll always beat him by a point or two, but I won't absolutely smash him (partly because he's getting bigger and better by the day). I want him to know what failure and struggle feel like. I want him to know what winning is about.

Because when that day comes – and it fucking will – when he beats me, I want him to enjoy it fully because he'll know what it's like to have started from the bottom. He'll know what it is to get steadily better and better at something. Those wins will feel far better when he thinks of all the failures he's endured on the way.

Being sacked by *SAS: Who Dares Wins* wasn't particularly pleasant. And yet it has left me even more hungry to succeed. Because I want to prove myself, and in the process get everyone who has doubted me, or slated me, or walked away from me to realise what a big mistake they made.

'Fuck you' is an amazing fuel.

LESSONS

Failure is the best teacher there is. When you open yourself up to failure, you'll super-charge your ability to learn and grow.

Never pass the buck, never point the finger. If you've crashed and burned, you've got to front up and take responsibility. Blaming others might make you feel better in the short term, but it also means you're never going to discover the amazing lessons that failure teaches us.

One step back, two steps forward. You might think failures are the end of something. But it's much better to think of them as steps on the way to success. Each failure brings your ultimate triumph a bit closer.

No setback is ever final. Don't let your failures define you or hold you back. What has happened to you isn't important. It's your response to it that people will remember.

Time is on your side. There's no need to rush. No matter what anybody else tells you, we've all got an abundance of time. So don't feel as if there's ever pressure to get things right first time or settle for things that fall short of your expectations. Try, fail, try again and fail better, until you get to where you want to be.

You can turn failures into opportunities. Setbacks can break apart old routines and make us see the world with new eyes. They give us the chance to start again and try new things, new ways of solving our problems. That's tremendously exciting.

CHAPTER 7

DON'T TELL LIES

Honesty is always, always the best policy.

WHEN I WAS in my first year at Portsmouth Grammar School, better known as PGS, I played a lot of football. This was when the money was flowing in the aftermath of my dad's death. I used to play for a Saturday team called Victory 86, I was part of the Southampton FC academy and I was captain of the school team. One week I trained with the academy on a Friday night after school, the next day I turned out in a match for Victory 86, and I was supposed to play for the school on Sunday. Quite frankly, however, I couldn't be arsed, despite being captain. I realise now how bad that sounds, but it was true. I'd lost my weekend and I had nothing left in the tank.

On Monday I was back at school. As I went from one lesson to another, Mr Nicholson, the PE teacher, collared me in the stairwell.

'Middleton, come here.'

'Yes, sir.' Aware that I'd let him down the day before, I shuffled reluctantly over to where he was standing.

'Where were you on Sunday? We lost, we didn't have our captain. What's going on?' He seemed angry – and hurt.

'Oh, sir, I went to Southampton on the Friday, I played for Victory 86 on the Saturday and I was too tired to play on Sunday.' I knew my excuse sounded unconvincing, but I didn't really know what else to say.

'Too *tired*? You're never too tired.' Mr Nicholson was having none of it, and I could see where he was coming from. I was a really active kid, the sort that never stopped moving. 'That's a load of rubbish. Young boy like you? Never in a million years. You're not going to be captain for our next game.'

He shot me a disappointed look, then stomped off. My sense is that he thought I'd be gutted to be relieved of the captaincy. But actually it didn't bother me at all. I was just pleased to have got away with such a light punishment. As soon as he'd disappeared from view I was ready to banish the whole thing from my mind. My day went on, I carried on going from class to class and then I went back home.

That night my mum was making tea and we started chatting.

'Did PGS say anything about you missing the game?'

'Yeah, Mr Nicholson confronted me and asked me why I hadn't turned up. He told me I should have played.'

'Really? He said that?'

'Yeah,' I could see that she was beginning to get defensive on my behalf. 'Then he sort of grabbed hold of my ear and pulled me down a flight of stairs and told me that they were stripping me of being captain next week.'

To this day I can't tell you why I decided to come out with such an extravagant lie. Maybe I was a bit more annoyed than I'd thought at the way Mr Nicholson had told me off. Maybe it was something in the tone of my mum's voice. Or maybe there was something inside me that just wanted to see what would happen. I don't know. When you're a kid, you do things that don't make much sense.

'He did *what*?'

I explained again. Mum was incandescent, and at just that moment my stepdad came in. The situation was escalating quickly. He'd overheard my conversation with Mum and was already fuming, which admittedly didn't take much.

'Right, I'm going straight over to the school in the morning and I'm going to fucking tell them that this is unacceptable.'

He got angry a lot. Sometimes he'd go out and do stuff, mostly it was just blowing off steam. At this stage I really didn't think anything would happen, so I went upstairs and played about for a bit.

Which, it turned out, was a serious mistake. The next morning the headmaster came up to me in the corridor and said, 'I want you in my office at the end of school.'

For fuck's sake, I thought. *What have I done now?* I'd thought so little of the lie I'd told that at that stage I hadn't made the link.

'Of course, sir. I'll see you then.'

When I walked into his office later that afternoon after the bell had gone I found my mum and stepdad waiting for me. I still hadn't clocked it.

'What the hell is all this about?' I said.

Then an angry, bewildered Mr Nicholson walked in. Right, I told myself, *this* is what it's all about.

My stepdad immediately went on the attack. Looking as if he could barely restrain himself, he said to the PE teacher: 'If you touch my son again I'll punch your fucking head through the wall. How would you like it if I grabbed *you* by the ear?'

Mr Nicholson didn't really react; he just glanced across at the headmaster, as if willing him to intervene.

A horrible sensation surged down my spine. Suddenly the room felt really hot. Shit. What had I done? But I couldn't help myself. It was easier to lie at this point than to tell the truth so I carried on with the same story, while my mum and stepdad kept fuelling the situation. Every angry comment they made, every threat they issued, seemed to make honesty that bit harder.

Mr Nicholson looked even more hurt and angry than he had the day before. He tried to look me in the eye but I kept my head down.

'I didn't touch you, did I?'

'Yes, you did. You pulled me by the ear and dragged me down the stairs.' I still couldn't meet his gaze.

Another intervention from my stepdad. 'My son's not a liar.'

The headmaster, clearly trying to keep control of a situation that was threatening to get out of hand, asked me if I understood how serious my accusation was.

'Yes, sir, but it did happen.'

At that moment my parents grabbed me and we all moved towards the door.

'I've had enough of this,' my mum said. 'You'll be hearing from us.'

I was off school for a whole week after that. Day followed day and I kept to my story. On Wednesday I asked when I'd be going back to PGS. Mum's answer came as a shock. 'You're not going back until the court case is over. Until then you can't be under the same roof as the teacher who assaulted you.' *Court case?* 'We're hiring lawyers, we're going to sue the school.'

Another couple of days went by. At the end of the week a man came to the house and the adults sat me down.

'Who's this?' I asked.

They explained that he was the lawyer who'd be looking after the court case.

'Before we go down this road,' the man said, 'this is your last chance to tell us what really happened. We need to know for absolute sure before we go any further. Suing a teacher and a school's a big deal. Now is the time to back out if we need to. Tell us the truth. We won't get angry, we won't tell you off. We just need to know. Did Mr Nicholson grab you by the ear and pull you down a flight of stairs?'

The lawyer had taken out a fountain pen, which was now hovering over an official-looking bit of paper. I knew then with absolutely certainty that as soon as he started writing that there would be no way back. I felt way out of my depth. *This is real*, I said to myself, *this is happening*. I had to make it stop.

'No.'

My voice was really small now. All I wanted was to disappear. I looked up. My stepdad was *raging*. He was desperate to go some. My mum shrugged it off more easily.

'Oh well,' she said, 'it doesn't matter anyway. That teacher's an arsehole.' Her instinct was always to stick up for me, no matter what I'd done.

I saw the rest of that term out, but at its end I was expelled. Me and PGS parted ways forever.

One small lie had ended up as a big, consequential lie. I realised how powerful they could be. And it had all been so frictionless. Those words had spilled so easily out of my mouth and could have ended up rearranging several lives. I think back now and am horrified about the impact it must have had on poor Mr Nicholson, and probably his family too. I put him through hell because I couldn't tell the truth. My mum and stepdad must also have been put through the ringer, not just through their concern when they believed I'd been attacked, but also the humiliation of discovering it had all been a fantasy. As for me, there were no real consequences. Nothing that I cared about at any rate.

If there's anybody from my past I'd like see again it would be Mr Nicholson. Thirty years on, I still feel as if I need to make amends.

YOU SHOULD ALWAYS tell the truth. In almost every single scenario I can imagine, it's a million times better to be honest than to slip into a lie. This should be the easiest of all the rules to follow. It might involve a small amount of immediate discomfort, but even this should be balanced out by the knowledge that the long-term benefits of honesty outweigh the short-term advantages you can occasionally gain by lying your arse off.

And yet lying is something people do despite their better nature. They might know in the rational part of their brain that it's always better to tell the truth, so why is it that they sometimes find it so hard to be honest? I've got good experience of this because I was brought up on lies. My mum was a compulsive liar. Looking back on it, she wasn't actually very good at it – I can now laugh about some of the fibs she used to tell – but she found it impossible to stop herself.

She was always trying to shape the world to suit her better, and if truth got in the way of that she never seemed to mind. She lied to get herself out of tough situations or to make herself look better. I'm not sure she even knew she was doing it.

But because I was a kid, I believed everything she said. I had no reason to doubt her. It meant that we all grew up cocooned by lies, so telling them became second nature to us. We just didn't know any better. Lies used to just roll off my tongue. I'd heard so many from my mum that none of my evasions or mistruths felt strange. There were times when I'd lie without thinking about it. I lied to get out of trouble, I lied even when I wasn't in trouble, and I lied during my first marriage, telling myself that the situation I was in wasn't just OK, it was actually just what I *wanted*.

It was only when I became an adult that I started to see my mum's lies for what they were and to properly understand the damage they could cause. I went from believing everything she said to believing nothing that she said.

Even so, I found lying a difficult habit to shake. It was something that I hated about myself, but I couldn't help myself. I had to make a concerted effort to stop. And now I've got a family of my own, it's the one thing I will not tolerate at home. If you let your children lie even once, a little voice in their heads will say, 'Oh, I've got away with that.' Whatever effort you've saved yourself right this second will be dwarfed by the trouble you've laid up for yourself in the future. Luckily my kids are terrible at lying – I can always tell when they're in the middle of one – but it annoys me that they'd even try!

THERE'S NOT MUCH advice I can give you about lies. Telling the truth doesn't demand hard work or practice. You can't exactly get *better* at telling the truth. All it requires is that you make a choice. It's a simple exertion of your will.

So this chapter will be unlike the others. I'm just going to outline the reasons why I think lying is a dead-end game. And then maybe, next time you're tempted to tell a lie, even a small one, you can bear them in mind. Maybe it will be enough to stop you.

LIES SOLVE NOTHING

Lying often seems like a good solution in a tricky situation. If somebody asks whether you've done something, you can just deny it, and then walk away scot-free.

Except that's not quite true. It's not even nearly true. Almost everyone who lies gets found out at some point. That might happen in the seconds after the words have passed your lips or it could be years later. You're still going to get caught, and you're probably still going to have to face up to the consequences. So why not get it over with? People respect honesty.

And let's say nobody realises you're fibbing. That's a win, right? Actually, no. You're creating a new reality based on that lie. That's what happened to me back when I was a kid. I thought I'd got away with it, but I realised I'd forced myself into a position where I was having to tell the same lie over and over again.

That distorted reality you create makes it harder to solve whatever situation prompted it. I'll always tell my kids, 'I'm here to sort out anything. Good or bad, I'll always be there to help them. If you lie to me, then my answer will be a lie, my solution will be a lie, and we'll get nowhere. You'll get found out. You'll look like an idiot. I'll look like an idiot. And the problem will still be there.'

LIES HURT

What started out as a tiny lie to get me out of trouble could have ended up ruining Mr Nicholson's career. God knows what might have happened to him if I hadn't finally admitted that what I'd initially claimed was untrue. When you lie you cause damage to other people. That should be enough by itself to stop you if you're ever tempted to be dishonest. When you're thinking of lying, take a moment to consider what impact your dishonesty might have on the other people involved.

But there are also consequences for the person who's telling the lies. It's not just that you're often left with a sense of guilt or shame about what you've done, and that the need to keep reinforcing your lies involves horrible psychological acrobatics. When you gain a reputation as a liar, it has all sorts of implications.

It can be small stuff that initially seems inconsequential. We've all had that mate who's always telling extravagant porkies about the things he's done ('I had a trial at Spurs') or his success with women ('I pulled six birds on holiday'). They're funny ... until they're not. Nobody respects them or takes them seriously – and they end up as a joke.

I saw at first-hand the impact my mum's lies had on her relationships with other people. It's so dangerous to be in the position where nobody trusts a single word that comes out of your mouth. It's corrosive on your personal and professional relationships. And it's horrible for everybody close to you. I loved my mum, I knew that she always had my best interests at heart, and yet I also knew that most if not all of the time she was lying her socks off.

After a while I pretty much stopped listening to her. She could talk for hours, and I'd take nothing in. What was the point? It was all lies. The thing that hurt me most were the lies she told about the circumstances of my father's death. I remember her telling me how horrendous it had been for her. She talked about waking up and doing CPR on him, and how blood had splattered out of his mouth and onto the mirrors. But she'd forgotten that I'd walked into their bedroom and saw my father lying prone on the bed surrounded by policemen. My memory of that moment is so vivid. There wasn't any blood. And her lies carried on from there, just a sequence of little things: well, that's not true, nor is that, nor is that. What about that? Nope, not true.

These lies cast a shadow over the last decade or so of her life. They damaged my relationship with her, they damaged her relationship with other people.

Do you really want to be the sort of person who nobody trusts? Do you want people to think that every word that spills from your mouth is a lie?

Finally, if you can't be honest with yourself, the only person you're cheating is you. If you blame other people for your own failures, tell yourself reassuring fibs to cover your own weaknesses and pretend that you're a different human being to the one you really are, you'll just end up living a lie. Day after day you'll be making a series of small bad decisions in order to support the big bad decision. Your existence will be wasted playing catch-up.

LESSONS

Lies don't work. You might be able to stay out of trouble for a little while by telling a lie, but your dishonesty will always catch up with you.

Lie beget lies. One lie leads to another. Then another. Then another. Before long, your whole existence will be a fabrication. Is that what you really want?

Lies can ruin lives. I could have destroyed my teacher's career if I'd been stupid or reckless enough to carry on pretending that he'd hurt me. If you're ever considering being dishonest, think of the effect it will have on other people.

Lies erode trust. People don't trust liars. They don't confide in them, they don't like them and they don't want to be around them.

CHAPTER 8

STOP WORRYING ABOUT THE FUTURE

How to cope with anxiety and even
make it work for you.

ANYBODY WHO CLAIMS they've never been anxious is a liar.

Sometimes you know anxiety is coming for you. You'll see it careering up the hallway, screaming at the top of its voice; it's not nice, but at least you have a chance to get yourself ready. At other times it can be a bit more insidious. One moment you're doing fine, the next you find that anxiety has crept up behind you and has already started dripping poison into your ear.

I'M NOT SURE I ever thought that life on civvy street would be exactly easy. But I probably did believe that since my days of life-or-death combat were behind me I wouldn't have much to feel anxious about. Which, of course, was absolute nonsense. What I learned very quickly is that the thing about anxiety is that the discomfort you feel rarely matches the size of the problem you're facing.

By the time I'd left the military my family was growing and so, suddenly, were my outgoings. Shyla and Gabriel were both really young, still only toddlers really. After years of being able to rely on a steady paycheque and a comfortable house at the barracks, I found I was having to bounce around Africa grafting my balls off just so we could rent somewhere half decent.

But I made progress, and after a while I could tell myself that I'd begun to build up a viable security business. I'd do a job here, a job there. I wasn't making bad money, and yet everything felt precarious. Always, at the back of my mind, there was this voice saying, *Where's your next job? What will you do after this one has finished? Why aren't you putting money aside for a rainy day? Do you think you're really good enough for this?*

On the outside I was the same old outgoing Ant, the life and soul of every party. Inside I was almost tearing myself to pieces with stress. More than anything, I didn't want to pass that angst or uncertainty on to my kids. It wasn't that I expected them to grow up eating caviar off gold plates, but I didn't want them to ever have to worry about money. I could remember only too well how strange and unsettling I'd found the lurches in my family's financial situation when I'd been a boy.

Nevertheless I was just about keeping everything together, and then the rainy day came, far sooner than I'd ever expected. First I got my fingers burned in a diamond deal that went wrong. I put too much trust in the wrong people, my investors demanded their money back and I was left with a big hole in my finances. Luckily, another job came up in South Africa. It was a good gig with a good wage; enough to get me back into the black with a decent amount to spare. I got on a plane, did the work, flew back and thought to myself, *Fine, I've got enough in my account to keep us going for two weeks, but I'm sure I'll get paid before then.* Two weeks came and went, and there was still no sign of the payment. Left without any other options, I did what I could to keep us afloat. I pawned my only nice watch, an Omega. The £800 I got for that lasted us another fortnight. Still no money. Worse, I'd nothing left I could use to raise more funds. We were, not to put too fine a point on it, absolutely fucked.

All day long, and in the last drawn-out seconds before I was finally able to sleep, all I could think about was that gap in my bank account. I couldn't concentrate on anything else. I should have been out there looking for new jobs. I should have been helping Emilie around the house. Instead, I brooded. I was constantly tense, and found myself snapping at Emilie and the kids. I look back now and ask myself, *What were you thinking?* And yet I was completely overwhelmed by anxiety. I could barely see around its edges.

One morning, after I'd stumbled blearily downstairs to the kitchen to fetch Gabriel's milk, I opened the fridge and found that the bottle was empty except for a tiny amount that might just have stretched to a cup of tea. Everyone else in the house was asleep. I stood there for a moment in the dark room, my face lit up by the fridge's artificial glow, feeling a deep helplessness that I'd never experienced before. It brought everything that had been nagging at me over the last months into sharp focus.

Don't get me wrong, we had food in the freezer and the family wasn't about to starve. But still, how had it got to the point where I didn't have the cash to buy my kid some milk? I crept upstairs, intending to see if Emilie maybe had some coins in her purse. It was only then that I remembered the little terramundi pot in Shyla's room. Emilie's sister had bought it for her, and Emilie and I had steadily given her coins to fill it up. I held it in my hands for a couple of seconds. It was maybe a quarter full. Even if most of the coins were 20ps – and I was pretty sure they would be – I knew there would be enough in there to at least buy a litre of milk.

At first I thought if I jabbed a knife in I might be able to coax some of the money out. Not a chance. Which led to Plan B: fuck it. I smashed the jar and, to my great joy, glinting dully amid the shards of broken piggy bank were a surprising number of £1 and £2 coins. There was maybe £60. Emilie had clearly been a good and busy fairy.

My excitement was followed first by one thought, *I never want to be in this situation again*; and then another, *I'll always find a way*. On the one hand, I was at maybe my financial rock bottom. I was raiding my daughter's piggy bank to find the money to pay for my son's milk! On the other, something had turned up. I'd worried and worried and worried about this moment, and what would happen when it came. That anxiety had taken a toll on me and also everybody around me. The fear of what *might* happen had been a kind of torture. And yet the worst thing had happened, and we were all still standing. The day began and we got on with things. Now that my mind had cleared I was able to start actively pursuing new jobs. A week later, the cheque came in.

THE WORLD OF 'WHAT IF?'

Lots of people who struggle with anxiety exist in one of two realms. They're either living in the past – gripped by the memory of a damaging experience – or they're living in the future, afraid of what *might* happen, exactly as I was, pacing around my house in Essex, worrying about how I was going to pay my next bill. I was more focused on what might happen than what was actually going on in front of me.

When you're living in the future instead of the present, then you're not really living in the real world at all. The future is all imagination, all potential. It's what you *think* is going to happen. You might be afraid of losing your house or job in the future, but until any of those things happen they're not real. They're a fantasy.

Similarly, the past is memory – it's another form of imagination. A lot of people end up floating in one of these two imaginary realms. They're either living in the past, which they can't change, or the future, which they can't predict. It's no wonder that they feel anxiety and stress!

The danger is that if you're not fully committed to the present, then you'll end up focusing on what doesn't yet exist at the expense of what's actually in front of you. In that period before I had to break into my daughter's piggy bank I'd have moments when I realised I was letting my anxiety about the future leach into my day-to-day work. I risked doing the sort of bad job that would have stopped me ever getting a contract again. Which, ironically, would mean that I'd have been complicit in making my fears come true.

Similarly, when we're doing tasks during *SAS: Who Dares Wins* that involve a helicopter flight beforehand, there will be some recruits who'll really be embracing the experience. They'll act a bit like those dogs that you see happily sticking their heads out of the window of a moving car. But there will also always be a couple cowering in the corner, unable to think about anything other than the challenge lying ahead of them. If I see that, I'll ask them, 'Have you ever been on a helicopter before?' They'll invariably say No, and my reply is always, 'So fucking *enjoy* it then. When are you going to have this chance again? You're sitting by the door. Look around you! Instead you've got your head down draining yourself while thinking about something that's still some way off in the future. Obsessing about it isn't going to make it go away.'

You can't let your fear of the future infect your enjoyment of the present. Whichever way you slice it, we're just not on this planet for long enough to spend our whole time worrying about worst-case scenarios. Don't overthink things. Don't jump into that water. Sweep the net in and grab what you need, but don't stay a second longer. Once you go too deep you'll start dragging up muck that belongs at the bottom of the sea.

When I say that, I'm not for a second denying the seriousness of anxiety. I know it's something that can have a profound impact on people; it can really tear them apart. And I have seen at first-hand how paralysing it can be. That voice in your head gets so loud, so insistent that it becomes a self-fulfilling prophesy. You get trapped by your fears, convinced there's no alternative.

But it doesn't need to be that way. I'm never going to be able to banish all those things – like money worries or impending job interviews – that make us feel anxious. What I can do is offer you some things that I've found useful in controlling anxiety. Who knows, you might even find a way to use this complex, uncomfortable emotion to your advantage.

THE FUTURE'S A MYSTERY, AND THAT'S OK

Life can change at the flick of a switch. I can still remember those occasions in Afghanistan when I went into compounds to take out a senior Taliban. After we'd captured or killed their husband, we'd often find the man's wife and kids in the next room. Suddenly we were confronted by human beings who had just lost a husband or father; in a matter of seconds their world had been smashed to pieces. Going to prison was another reminder of how fragile the existences we build ourselves can be. A moment of stupidity meant that I almost lost everything.

And yet that sort of lightning bolt can be positive too. The call from the producers of *SAS: Who Dares Wins* came completely out of the blue, and it set me on an unbelievable trajectory.

The point is that the future is chaotic and uncertain and pretty much impossible to predict. For some people that's the source of their anxiety. I find it unbelievably exciting. Once you accept that you can't predict the future, you'll be liberated.

It's precisely because so much of the future is unknown that I don't spend too much time planning my life. You can get so obsessed by a set of fixed goals that you let other, far better opportunities pass you by.

If I'd planned my future meticulously, then it's likely that when I got that call asking me if I was interested in having a meeting about a show that might or might not get commissioned for Channel 4, I'd have turned round and said that I was focusing on building my security business. I'd have missed out on *SAS: Who Dares Wins*.

This isn't to say that you should completely abandon planning or precautions. But you have to remember that there's always a limit to what you can do. You can put savings away, you can take insurance out. What you can't do, however, is anticipate in minute detail what will actually happen.

What's also really damaging is that so many people have an in-built assumption that their future is inevitably going to be full of disaster; that what's coming down the line is worse than what they're facing now. This seems mad to me. Why not be excited? Why not think about the possibility that the future might be bringing you untold riches? I've come to realise that it's unhealthy to spend my days planning what I'd do in worst-case scenarios. Why would I want to be in that headspace?

You have to trust the process, and your own abilities. More often than not you'll be equal to even the worst that life can throw at you.

CONTROL WHAT YOU CAN, IGNORE WHAT YOU CAN'T

Anxiety can be a complex, confusing and disempowering emotion. It convinces you that you're in the hands of fate, that there's not much you can do to affect your future.

At the same time, paradoxically, it can make you feel responsible for stuff that's out of your control. You end up working yourself into the ground, making yourself fucking miserable, for something you know you'll never be able to achieve.

The antidote to this is to be ferociously clear about what aspects of your personal and professional life you can and can't control. Whenever you can feel that prickle of anxiety rising up your spine, try to think as clearly as you can about the situation. What's in your gift to change? What can you do to prepare? And what's completely out of your hands?

Why spend the two hours before you have an interview letting yourself get eaten up by anxiety? Why not try to conserve that nervous energy and make it work for you later instead of letting it hollow you out right now? Have you worked hard? Have you prepared for the interview? Well then, what are you worried about? You'd be quite right to be anxious if you've just dossed about. That's fucking on you. You can either sort that problem out or, if it's too late, learn the lesson. But if you've properly prepared, then you're good to go and there's no need to worry.

My income dips and soars. That's always going to happen if you're self-employed. It means that occasionally I get the taxman coming after me with a bill that I'm not in a position to settle, perhaps because I'm waiting for payment for something. Very quickly, I've found, they resort to sending you shitty letters. Maybe once upon a time that would have sent me into an anxious spin. Now my response has become: *If I don't have the fucking money to pay it, then I ain't got the fucking money to pay it. What do you want from me?*

I don't stress about it because there's nothing I can do. Relax. Don't worry. It's going to get done. Maybe not soon enough for the person who's going mad chasing me. But it will get done. Ultimately, I can only do the best that I can do. If I've done everything possible, in good faith, why stress about things? If someone's asking for something that I can't give them, then why should I take that angst onto my shoulders?

Sometimes the best I can do won't be good enough. And I can live with that. Focus on what's in your grasp. Treat everything else as noise and nonsense.

IT'S NOT THE END OF THE WORLD

Part of being able to shed anxiety is making your peace with the idea that things will sometimes go wrong – when they do, the chances are that not only will you survive, but you'll come out the other end stronger.

That's why I think it's so important that you don't catastrophise. You might think that losing your job will be a complete disaster, but it probably won't be that bad. You don't know, that change in your circumstances could lead to better things. Even if it doesn't, however, you'll find a way of getting by. One of the things that helped when I was agonising over building my protection business was reminding myself that even if I did stop getting high-paid jobs in exotic countries, there would always be a way to provide for my family. I knew that I could have got a steady gig as a protection officer in London: £150 a day to guard an Arab family or a pop star. If I had to empty bins to make some money, then fine, I'd go and empty bins.

Most of us are going to live long lives and still be working into our seventies. In that context, a single setback doesn't matter too much. Everyone will have plenty of chances to pick themselves up and try again. (See Chapter 6 on failure and Chapter 12 on resilience for further advice on how to cope when life doesn't go according to plan.)

NOTHING ENDURES

The other thing about the incident with my daughter's piggy bank was that after I'd carefully stuck it all back together and replaced the coins I didn't tell anybody else, not even Emilie, what had happened for another couple of years. By that time my life had changed completely. And that's the strange thing. When I look back at the surge of panic I experienced when I saw that not only had we run out of milk but that I didn't even have the money to buy more, it feels almost ridiculous. How could I have got so worked up? This emotion that felt so all-consuming at the time has become just another anecdote.

If you can, try to remind yourself that whatever now seems big and terrifying won't last. Nothing, however awful it might seem, goes on forever. Everything comes to an end.

LAUGHTER FIXES (ALMOST) EVERYTHING

Anxiety can sometimes feel a bit like somebody's cast a spell over you. You're in its grip and it can seem as if there's nothing you can say or do that will lift it. All the rational and carefully considered arguments you try just seem to melt away as soon as they come into contact with anxiety's strange magic.

I've always found that humour, even dark humour, can help break that spell. In the midst of viciously tense moments, a joke can help relax everybody and create instant bonds. More than that, it takes you outside of yourself and allows you to see the whole situation from a different perspective.

VIRAL ANXIETY

A lot of the time the greatest stress comes from outside. One moment you're feeling fine, the next there's someone in your ear saying, 'Ant, you need to do this, you need to do that.' Suddenly your head is full of another person's demands and needs.

Anxiety and stress breed anxiety and stress – they're so contagious. One anxious person in a room is enough to set the nerves jangling of everybody else in there with them. There's enough stress and anxiety in the world without you generating more for other people. If you're feeling stressed and anxious, be aware of the effect that you can have on other people. By the same token, if you know you're predisposed to stress and anxiety, then keep your distance from people you know who generate these emotions. There are some anxious people out there who are never happier than when they've managed to dump a bit of that anxiety on you. Why open yourself up to that?

This is especially important because both stress and anxiety have become increasingly prevalent in recent years. There's a more anxious tone to our conversations and we feel more stressed about everything. Technology and social media have probably got quite a lot to answer for. But I also think the steady erosion of our freedom has contributed to the increasingly tense atmosphere that surrounds us. Our lives have become more regulated and controlled, and that inevitably creates an all-pervasive sense of anxiety in many of us.

It might only be in the background, and yet it's always there. I think perhaps the powers-that-be want people to be stressed and worried, because anxious people are easier to control. Paradoxically, it's understanding how restricted we really are that liberates us. If you want to live a freer, less anxious life, refuse to bow down to that pressure and control and take back charge of who you are. (See Chapter 3 on being authentic and Chapter 14 on the power of saying No for more advice on this subject.)

POSITIVE ANXIETY, POSITIVE STRESS

Something that isn't always given much attention is that both anxiety and stress can at times be positive. You can use them as emotions to help drive you on. Anxiety can just be a fear of not being good enough, of not operating to your maximum capacity. It sounds negative, but that's something you can flip into a positive. It doesn't need to inhibit you; instead it can provide the motivation you need to push yourself that bit harder. It's just your inner self pointing out the gap between where you are and where you should be. Many of the world's greatest sporting stars actually thrive on anxiety. The fear that they might get dropped from their teams or beaten by their rivals fuels a constant desire to improve and to perform at the highest level possible. Anxiety, for them, is the antidote to complacency.

The reason I do what I do is to try to protect my children and loved ones from the stresses and strains of life. That, I believe, is my responsibility as an adult and a parent. It also gives me a positive motivator. I know *why* I'm taking that aggravation onto my shoulders. I'm drawing on it to push myself on.

LESSONS

Don't get trapped in the world of 'what if?' We can't predict the future. We can't change the past. So work hard to live in the moment.

Work out what is and isn't in your hands. Use your time and energy to focus on what you *can* control. Don't dwell on what you *can't* control.

Remember that nothing endures. Try to take the long view. Whatever you're going through now won't last forever. It will soon be little more than a memory.

The future is bright. Free yourself of the assumption that the future is littered with trouble and strife. It's just as likely that it will contain exciting opportunities.

The power of humour. Laughter can be a brilliant antidote to stress and allows you to get a new perspective on your situation. No matter how bleak things seem, see if you can find a way to see the funny side.

Anxiety is a negative form of energy, but you can flip it into a positive. If you're worried that you're not in good enough shape for that marathon you've got coming up, use that anxiety to drive you on in your training.

CHAPTER 9

LEARN TO LOVE
YOUR BODY

**How to feel strong, feel happy and resist the
pressure to look like someone else.**

WHEN I WAS in the SBS I was going on missions so shrouded in secrecy that the government often refused to confirm that they had even taken place. I lived a shadowy existence. When I was on tour we were almost completely cut off from the rest of the world, and at times it was hard to believe that anything lay beyond the filth and danger of the mission. Months would go by without Emilie or anybody else who loved me knowing what I was doing, or where I was. Even when I was back at home in our little house at the barracks there would be nights when I would get a call just as we were sitting down to dinner. Within minutes I'd be gone. I could tell my family nothing about what I was about to do. It was jarring and uncomfortable. Sometimes it was heartbreaking. But that was my life and I could imagine no other.

If you'd crawled up to me on one of those long, freezing nights I spent shitting in a bag on surveillance and told me that within a few years I'd be on the front cover of a national magazine I'd have shit myself laughing and told you to fuck off. If you'd gone on to say that not only would I be on the cover of a magazine, but that I'd be topless, I'd have marched you to the doctor to get your head checked out.

But life is a funny old thing.

I DID MY first shoot for *Men's Health* in 2019. It was after that first rush of fame, when I was out there on a number of shows but still running day-camps. I was on my way to becoming well known, but not quite a celebrity.

So it was a surprise – a pretty good one – when they told me they wanted me on the cover. *Great!* I thought. That's when stuff got a bit more complicated, as I was inundated with offers from people offering to help me get really cut up for the photographs. It was all genuine, it was all meant kindly. But I just thought, *No.* I told them as politely as I could that while I appreciated their offers, I didn't think I needed to look any different. As I saw it I was extremely fit, not least because a good number of the recruits on *SAS: Who Dares Wins* were pretty much half my age – I had to keep myself in good nick so that they wouldn't embarrass me. I felt good in myself. What else would anybody want?

Well, it turns out, that wasn't enough. Nobody ever came out and said, 'Ant, you look shit, we need you to get shredded.' The pressure was more subtle than that. 'Ant, you've got eight weeks to get ready.' 'Ant, you've got four weeks to get ready.' 'Ant, you've got two weeks to get ready.' What did they want me to do? I'm not doing special training for a fucking *photoshoot*. Exercise is part of my lifestyle. I'll make adjustments according to any given situation, but I didn't want to throw it all out of the window just for the sake of a few photos. Nor was I willing to deplete my body of nutrients in the name of a crash diet. Fine for professional athletes or bodybuilders training for a specific event, but I was neither.

Do boxers look in unbelievable shape when they stand there for their weigh-ins? Yes. I've got so much respect for the discipline involved in getting to that position. But are they physically in a good place? No fucking way. Their bodies are screaming at them. You couldn't look like that 24/7. More to the point, you *shouldn't*.

I knew that I could really beast myself if I'd wanted to, do all the tricks, exist on a diet of creatine and low-fat water or whatever the fuck it is you need to do. And if I did that, I'd certainly look the part.

But the reason I didn't was stubbornness as much as anything else. I wanted to be true to myself and the way I lived. I hadn't signed up to presenting the world with a false, unrealistic picture of who I was. As far as I was concerned, that was that.

The shoot came and went, and to be honest I didn't really think about it very much. I didn't hear anything from them afterwards, but I just assumed it was normal. In fact the next message I got was one from them saying, 'Ant, here's the front cover, it's being published tomorrow, it's already been printed, blah, blah blah.'

The photograph was one that had been taken of me walking off set. I wasn't posing, I didn't have my arms back or anything and my shoulders were slumped. It was horrendous. My first thought was, *Fucking hell, don't I get a say in which photos they use?* I didn't know at the time what any of the other shots looked like, but it seemed to me as if they'd deliberately picked the worst one of me that they possibly could. My second thought was to worry whether I'd said or done something wrong at the shoot. Had I accidentally stolen another guy's sandwich? Was this their revenge?

I called them back in horror. 'What's going on?' I wasn't that bothered about how other people might react to the pictures, but I did think, *You cheeky fuckers*.

THE MAGAZINE HIT the shelves, followed by the predictable chorus of absolute no-marks speculating about my high body fat ratio or whatever those morons care about. Fine. *Men's Health* did what they did to get that precise reaction. The more their magazine got talked about, the more sales they made.

I told them that I only wished they'd run the whole thing by me. It could have been a brilliant opportunity to talk about body positivity. And that was it, we all moved on to other things. A couple of months later I got a call from my agent.

'Your edition was the bestselling *Men's Health* that year. You even beat David Beckham! How do you feel about doing another one next year? They're really keen to get you on the cover again.'

This seemed pretty funny to me.

'Ah, do they now?'

'They're going to give you approval over everything. In fact, they want you to be guest editor. You can come into the office, pick the photo you want to use. The whole lot.'

Cool, I thought. *This feels really exciting.* I followed up with a slightly spikier sentiment. 'I'm still not going to shred up. But I'll make sure that I stay on my game. And no more snaps taken in unguarded moments.'

This time round I was maybe half a stone lighter. I wasn't quite as busy, so I had a bit more time to train. And I looked amazing. I was really made up, because it was a representation of how I actually looked rather than a snapshot of me after having spent a week desperately trying to squeeze water out of my body. It showed me just as I was. I don't live in a gym. I don't live on a diet. I don't want to waste my life doing those things. Nor should you. But what I'll tell you is that I was far fitter when I posed for that first cover than I was for the second. I felt better and stronger then, I was closer to my natural weight. The Ant Middleton in 2019 would have had his 2020 equivalent for fucking breakfast.

* * *

WHEN I WAS a soldier I had to be in insane shape to do the job I did. It wasn't about looking good. Nobody was bothered whether or not there was a six-pack underneath my combat gear. They cared about whether I had enough stamina to keep going without sleep for three days straight. There was a level at which my body was required to perform, and it was my professional responsibility to ensure that it could. A toned body was never going to stop a bullet.

I've carried that attitude into civilian life. I look after myself because I want to feel good. I like waking up knowing I've not been eating shit food or putting alcohol or other poisons in my body. I like it that when I wake up and take a deep breath I can feel my lungs fill with air. If I don't get that sense of my lungs expanding, I'll go for a run.

More generally, I tailor what sort of exercise I take according to what I've got coming up. You don't exercise just to get stacked. You do it because you also want to feel confident and good in yourself.

If I know that there's filming for something like *SAS: Who Dares Wins* coming up, where I'm going to need to be nimble on my feet, I'll probably aim to lose a bit of bulk. So my exercise will include more cardiovascular stuff like running, rowing and swimming, and I'll replace weights with circuits.

As the summer approaches I might want to get a bit bigger and bulkier. It's nice to be able to chuck the kids around in the swimming pool, and who doesn't want to look good on the beach? So I'll cut down on the CV and hit some weighted circuits or some iron.

Ultimately, you should be looking to choose the body that's right for you, not the one that you think society expects you to have. Your body is your body. It's fucking unique. Love it. Be you. Don't be a fat cunt, but celebrate who and what you are. The problem is, I realise, that it's much easier said than done.

MAKE PEACE WITH YOUR IMPERFECTIONS

I've always been happy in my own body. The biggest reason for that is that I've made peace with my imperfections. When I look in the mirror I'll see stuff that I know isn't ideal and I'll have days when I get down about certain things.

But there's a clear difference between things you can and can't change. Work out what they are. Some mornings, I'll look at myself and think that maybe I could do with losing a bit of weight from around my stomach, or building up the muscle on my legs. That's stuff I can achieve without much fuss. I just need to alter the way I exercise for a bit. What I know I can't change is my height. I'm not short, but nor am I anybody's idea of tall. That's something that I'm absolutely fine with. And yet even if I wasn't, there's not much I could do, short of being stretched on a rack. Of course, I could be one of those men who try to steal a couple of centimetres here and there by wearing inserts in my shoes. But how much difference would that really make? I'd be spending my life trying to hide part of myself.

What I will say, and I cannot stress this enough, is that if any given procedure or activity is going to cost you your health in any way, shape or form, then it's not worth it. Steer clear, accept it and move on. It's madness to compromise your well-being for the sake of something small. Your health and your body aren't separate.

That's clearly true of risky cosmetic procedures. But it's also true of less dramatic stuff. If the shoes you're wearing are absolutely killing you, then you're probably not going to look that sexy when you walk into a room. If you go on a faddy diet to shift some weight but you're utterly miserable because you're living on carrot soup, is it really worth it? Especially since you're probably going to fall for the classic mistake of reaching your goal, then falling back into bad habits, and bang, before you know it, you're exactly where you started.

Be honest with yourself. And don't put too much pressure on cosmetic changes to change your life. Are you really unhappy because you're overweight? Or is it something else? Will losing a few pounds satisfy you, or will you just find another thing to try to change?

YOUR BODY, NOT OTHER PEOPLE'S

Men and women are both subject to incredible pressure to look a certain way. Men's magazines are as full of lads with ripped torsos as women's magazines are packed with impossibly thin girls. I know how easy it is to feel pressure to be something other than you are when you see photographs.

But the worst thing you can do is to fall into the trap of wanting to be somebody else. If somebody has achieved things by looking a certain way, or saying certain things, then great. Good for them. Learn lessons from them, sure, but don't imitate them. Don't try to walk the *exact* same path as them, no matter how much you want it. However hard you try, you're never going to be that person. You fit 100 per cent in your own skin, while you could probably force yourself into fitting 80 per cent into somebody else's. Even if you could somehow get to 90 per cent, you're still wasting 10 per cent of yourself, of your own potential, of the things that make you special. And why would you ever want to do that? (For more advice, see Chapter 2 on building self-confidence and Chapter 3 on being authentic.)

Remember that it's only you – ultimately – who has the answers. Physical trainers and therapists can both provide absolutely crucial guidance, but you'll know when you wake up in the morning whether you need to do something to sort your body out. It's communicating with us all the time. If your knees hurt, then that's your body telling you that you need to rest them. (See Chapter 4 on lifestyle for more information on listening to your body's needs.)

You fit into your skin for a reason, you're in your body for a reason. Be proud of it.

DON'T LET TROLLS RULE YOUR LIFE

The internet has made things even more complicated. Instagram, for example, is a curated fantasy that almost seems designed to make people feel worse about themselves. Those people who have abused their bodies for the sake of a photo that 99.9 per cent of the world will have forgotten even exists in a month's time are in a bad headspace. They can't wait for it all to be over so that they can go back to normal.

It also possible – in fact it's highly likely – that their photos have been Photoshopped to within an inch of their lives. That's not how any of these people look as they go about their daily lives.

But what causes even more harm are the cesspit-dwelling lowlife who exist only to denigrate other people. Even if you're not on social media you'll know the damage they do. There's the horrific sexist and racist abuse they inflict on so many people – both in and out of the public eye. And there's also the relentless drip, drip of their negativity. They lurk around people's mentions, waiting for an opportunity to tell somebody who they almost certainly haven't met that they're fat, their nose is too big or their skin is too dark. And fuck the consequences! They think that if you're offended, it's *your* problem.

I sometimes reflect on how lucky I've been that my success arrived when I was a grown man who'd had time to live with his body and appearance, and become secure in both. I know what's real, I know what's not. A kid who breaks through now is just going to be mentored by trolls. They'll be making life decisions based on the warped opinions of negative people. I mean, we live in a world where people were recently having a go at fucking Captain Tom. How is this happening? How is it even real?

What you need to remember is that people troll other people because they can. It's nothing to do with you or your achievements, and everything to do with their boredom and inadequacy. That they're *choosing* to do this in their free time says everything.

There's nothing you can ever say or do that will make them stop. And if you give in once, if you've internalised the voices of other people rather than embracing your own, then it'll never end. You'll always find a fault.

So why would you allow your sense of yourself to be governed by an arsehole with a keyboard and a negative mentality? It's almost liberating to know that you can't please everyone. It's only when you understand this that you can start living a more unfettered life where you aren't constantly looking over your shoulder. Your decision to say something, or wear something, should depend on the answer to two questions: a) does it give me pleasure? and b) does it hurt anybody? If it's yes to a) and no to b), go for it. The opinions of a sad-sack cunt who's still living in his mum's spare room shouldn't ever figure in your calculations.

LOOK AFTER YOURSELF

There's no shame in wanting to look well groomed, well looked-after. It's not shallow, it's not a waste of time. It's an important element in feeling positive about your body and general appearance.

When you're taking care of your appearance you're demonstrating that you're somebody who's worth that effort. Think about how good it feels to put on a crisp, clean shirt, or the sensation you get just after you've had your hair cut. That will translate into how you're perceived by others. If you can't be bothered to treat yourself properly, why should they?

But one question you should always be asking yourself is: who do you want to look good for? If the answer is anybody apart from yourself, then you're barking up the wrong tree.

ONE FINAL THING

We take so much for granted in our lives. Sometimes I think we forget how incredible our bodies are. We're entranced by the processing power of our new iPhone or the cool things an app can do, yet we forget that every day of life is a fresh miracle.

Everything we do on this planet is supported by these amazing machines that make 25 million new cells every second, whose bones are pound for pound stronger than steel, that can create new life. In the hours when we're awake, our brains produce enough energy to power a light bulb. It makes me sad to think that anybody could have a dysfunctional or uncomfortable relationship with something that's a source of so much wonder to me. When you're feeling low, when your mind is full of all the things you wish you could change about your body, try to remember how much it's capable of. My body, your body, everyone's bodies – they're all incredible.

LESSONS

Your body is amazing and unique. Cherish it. Celebrate the things that make your body different from anybody else's.

No body is ever perfect. Everyone has parts of their physique that they dislike. Work out what you can change, make peace with the things you can't change.

You fit 100 per cent into your own skin. Learn as much as you can from other people, but never try to imitate them.

Your health is paramount. There's no cosmetic improvement that justifies compromising your physical or mental well-being.

Internet trolls are inadequate leeches. They feed off attention, so don't give it to them.

Don't be ashamed of taking care of yourself. Wear nice clothes, get fancy haircuts, go to salons. Do whatever makes you feel happy. Just make sure that you're doing it for your benefit, not other people's.

CHAPTER 10

MAKE STRONG CONNECTIONS

How to have good relationships.

I LEFT MY first wife Hayley just as I was leaving the army. At the time we were living with our young son in married quarters in Aldershot. Amid the confusion and sadness that came with abandoning – or so I thought at the time – my dream of making a career as a soldier, I'm not sure I'd noticed how toxic our relationship had become. There was no trust between us, and whatever had first drawn us together had long since disappeared. Our life together had decayed into an unpleasant series of ugly arguments. But I put a lot of the friction and rows down to our particular circumstances. After all, our boy was only a few months old and I was going through a major change in my career. In fact, I was probably going through a major change in my personality.

The actual break came when I went up to London for all the tests you have to take before entering the Met Police. I'd had all the physical tests and endured the rough, tough final interview. They'd given me a start date, and I was elated to be make such positive steps forward after the bitterness and disappointment of the last few months.

It was pretty late by the time all that was over, so I ended up stopping off at my uncle's house in Wood Green for a cup of tea. I was so desperate to share my good news. I was still excited as I talked to him. 'I'll be able to see so much more of you,' I was saying. At that moment my wife called.

'Where are you?' No small talk, no 'How are you?'

'Oh, I'm just at my uncle's,' I said. Then I told her the good news. I thought she might be a bit pleased for me. After all, this was the start of something fresh and exciting for our whole family.

Instead, all I got was, 'Why the fuck have you stopped off at your uncle's?'

'Aren't you happy with the news?' I couldn't hide the hurt in my voice.

There was a brief silence, then she went back on the attack. 'But why are you still in London? Why didn't you come home to tell me first?'

That knocked me for six. I gathered myself and told her, quite honestly, that it was because she was at work. The conversation wasn't going well. It became even worse when I told her I was planning to stay the night at my uncle's. Then something snapped inside me. I didn't feel anger, but I seemed possessed by an amazing clarity and understood immediately what I needed to do. My nature is to be bubbly, happy and cheerful. And yet I found that lately I'd started to dread going home because I knew that as soon as I stepped through the door I'd become a different person

– a miserable, controlled shadow of who I really was. I'd somehow convinced myself that life was just about drudgery. You get up, go to work, come home again. Rinse and repeat.

My first wife was a good person and would go on to be a great mother to our son. But she was the wrong person for me. We didn't share the same values, we didn't have the same ambitions, we didn't have any real kind of connection. None of that had been obvious when we first met, and the all-consuming nature of army life had masked the chasm that had grown between us.

'I can't do this anymore,' I told her. My voice was firm, not betraying the emotion that had started to swell inside me. 'There's something wrong with you. There's something wrong with us. Do you know what, I'm not coming back. For good. Not ever.'

My uncle was sitting beside me as I talked with my wife. He looked up at me and nodded. That was the affirmation I needed. I knew I'd done the right thing.

That was it. I went back once, to sign the house over. Otherwise I was true to my word. I told her she could keep everything. It wasn't just a marriage I was ending, I was breaking up a family. Oakley wasn't much more than three months old at the time. I offered to take him, but in the end we agreed he'd live with her.

Hayley and Oakley moved back to Portsmouth with her mum, and for six months I stayed at my uncle's, working in a Wetherspoons in Wood Green while I waited to start my police training.

It was an instant decision, but I knew with overwhelming certainty that I had to make it. In the short term, however, there would be chaos and upset and hard work. We'd made a mistake, that much was clear. There was no proper bond between us. We were fundamentally incompatible people who'd managed to ignore those difference for long enough to exchange rings and bring a child into the world. And yet that wasn't enough. I'd have been miserable if we'd tried to stumble on. We'd all have been miserable if we'd carried on like that, just sleepwalking into creating a cruel, angry environment in which to raise our son. It wouldn't have been good for any of us.

In the weeks that followed I thought a lot about what had happened and why. We'd never really had a proper connection. We hadn't spent time talking to each other about what mattered to each other. Instead we'd gone from flirting with each other, to sleeping with each other, to getting aboard a plane to Cancún to get married, even though we probably both knew that we were doing the wrong thing.

I made two promises to myself then. The first was that I'd never be stupid enough to get married again. I remember thinking, *If this is what married life is like, then fuck me, count me out.* That didn't quite turn out according to plan, which of course is a very good thing. The second was that

I'd only let people into my life with whom I had a strong connection – human beings whose energy I responded to. I wasn't immediately successful at this. It's difficult to make those bonds when you're still working out who you are. So, I've made lots of missteps along the way, I've spent too much time with people who weren't worth it, and yet I've come out the other side. Two decades on, I think I've finally managed to keep that promise.

THE ONE THING YOU CAN'T FAKE

The earth is one big energy ball, the source of incredible amounts of power. There's an energy from the earth that runs through us, helping our hearts beat, making trees grow.

I'm not interested in hippy bullshit. You're not going to see me talking about chakras or trying to sell healing water. You'll never see Ant Middleton in a kaftan, beads or a tie-dye T-shirt.

But I am spiritual in the sense that I feel connected to the world. When you have that connection to the planet and yourself, there's not much that you feel you can't do, there's not much that you won't try and there's even less that you won't achieve. There are so many positive repercussions: your senses will be heightened, your energy will increase, you'll find it easier to establish meaningful relationships and your existing relationships will be improved.

There's one moment I always remember that crystallised a lot of this for me; it was one of those epiphanies you sometimes get. I saw that if you strip everything else away, we're standing on a ball of energy. We were filming *SAS: Who Dares Wins* in Chile. The moment itself came when we were doing the recces around the mountains. All around us were these huge fields of scree, the loose pieces of rock that collect on the sides of mountains and hills following rockfall. It's the mountain cutting its toenails, pushing all the shit and debris down its flanks, just as we do with our own bodies when we shed all the material that we no longer need or want. It made me think, *These mountains are moving.*

As I was walking along, trying to process what I was seeing, I heard an enormous noise, almost like an explosion, followed by a ringing echo. My first thought was, *What the fuck is this?* The mountains to my left were a good five or six hundred metres away and they had hurled a piece of slate that was maybe two foot long within inches of my fucking head. I ducked and looked round as it sliced through the air behind me. If its trajectory had been only very slightly different, it would have taken my head clean off.

To me it was like the mountain was putting on a performance to demonstrate its impossible strength. I felt it was saying, 'You're right, Ant, I am fucking amazing. Now watch *this*.' We'd been warned about the mountain before we'd set off. Now I knew why.

It left me awed.

Energy has to go somewhere. Everything gets regenerated. What do you think happens to the energy stored in your body when you die? The idea that 'we're only here for a visit' seems so way off for me. We're *part* of everything that goes on around us. We're not tourists. We're as important to the planet as it is to us.

Now clearly, I'm not thinking about the planet's mysteries as I go about my daily life. But that sense of connection informs so much of what I do. I'm a strong believer in the importance of energy in our lives. Human beings are just like that mountain – we're all constantly giving off energy; in fact we're fizzing and popping with it. Sometimes that energy is positive, sometimes it's negative. If the energy inside me is bad, then people are going to feel that. You can smile as much as you want, but you can't fake positivity.

I can go into a room and there'll be someone there just pumping out negative vibes. Now, they can pretend that they're positive all day long, they can swear to me on their kids' lives that they're a positive person, but I'll know different. I can tell if they're hiding behind a counterfeit persona. You can't fake energy.

Once you know to look for it, you can sense jealousy and envy. You can sense the little things people say and do to try to protect themselves. My senses will give me a good idea of whether I want to be around, or work with, the person they really are rather than the person they claim to be. It's the equivalent of that moment when you sense somebody standing beside your bed *before* you wake up.

Connection is so crucial, both in your private and professional lives. I don't mean the superficial connection that comes with small talk about the weather or football or whatever it is that comes out of our mouths when we want to fill space but don't know what to say. I mean proper, deep connections. Where two people share values and aspirations and trust. They're the sorts of human being I want to surround myself with.

I knew that Emilie was the right person for me as soon as we met. We formed an immediate connection. And yet it was also one of those situations where you have to look a bit below the surface. You don't just go by what someone says, or where they go, or what they wear. That's mostly just froth. What you should really be paying attention to is the energy they give off. It's why I'll never pay too much attention to somebody else's judgement about another person. I want to be able to make my mind up. I trust my senses more than I ever would another human being's opinion.

QUALITY NOT QUANTITY

I've got to the point where the quantity of people that I interact with doesn't interest me. What's important is the quality. I've cut away the hangers-on, the acquaintances.

They're just flotsam and jetsam, who, if you're not careful, will try to drag you in the wrong direction. My rule now is: if you don't benefit my life, if all you bring is drama and useless chitchat, then I don't have time for you.

So I know that I'm probably not the friend I used to be. I'm very aware of that.

I don't have the time to make those little calls where you catch up with your mates and find out how they're doing. I don't have people round my house. I never go out now. I've done my drinking, I've done my partying, I've done my fighting. Those things might have brought me fleeting pleasure, but they left me in the void. They were a way of filling my time, not using it. When I think back to those days I just see somebody who was in cruise control, somebody motoring along trying to please other people who I didn't understand, and who didn't really understand me.

I'm someone who always wants to give 100 per cent. So if I know I can only be 50 per cent of the friend my mates need, I'd rather not do it. A bit of me isn't any better than none of me. When I did give 100 per cent to my friends it meant I was only half the father and husband I needed to be. It left me in prison because of a fight somebody else started. Or it meant I was hungover when I should have been with my kids.

I want to be surrounded by people with whom I have strong, meaningful connections, whose presence benefits me. I'm not talking about money or material things. What's important to me is that you're super-positive, funny and supportive. The few friends I do still see I regard more as family. They're an extra gang of brothers and I'd do anything for them. They're people who push me to succeed and to be better. They make me hungry. It's an ecosystem in which we all work for each other. But if you're outside that ecosystem then I'm not interested.

Don't forget that finding people with whom you can form strong connections isn't necessarily about searching for human beings who are your exact replica. My best friend, whom I met when we passed Selection together, couldn't be any different from me. He's still in the military – sergeant major now – and he's never going to leave. He's also so antisocial that he wouldn't even go into a shop to buy jeans over the counter. He's an introvert, the idea of talking to other people horrifies him, and yet we get on like a house on fire. That's because we connect on the things that are really important.

THE MOST IMPORTANT CONNECTION OF ALL

Emilie is beautiful. Half of Essex was after her. She was out and about, she liked to have fun and she could have been mistaken for a bit of a party girl. And yet beneath that it was immediately clear that we had the same values. She's lovely to be around and has an easy-going energy. But I could also sense her integrity and loyalty. I could sense that she respected herself. I could sense that she was a lovely, genuine person. That all-important connection was there.

As the years have gone by it's got better and better. I love loving her. I enjoy the way we've changed over time – how we challenge and improve each other. I'm a better person because of the role she has played in my life. I hope she would say the same about me.

Partnership is so important. You have to find someone that's compatible. This seems obvious, but there are people out there who would prefer to have somebody who looks good on their arm than somebody they're connected to. They'll all end up making the same mistake I did and enter into a relationship with a person they think looks nice. For the first few months they can play happy, ignoring what they know to be true: they're not compatible. A month goes by, or a year, or five years and then they realise it's too late. They might have got married, or had kids. It gets to the point where to end that relationship will cause all kinds of collateral damage. Don't be the kind of fool who puts more thought into the brand of vacuum cleaner they buy than what sort of person they're going to spend the rest of their life with.

The best relationships are those where the two parties have been honest from day one. You'll only be able to make proper connections with others if you've already made that connection with yourself. If you're pretending to be somebody else, you're never going to form meaningful bonds with others – because you'll all be participating in a pantomime of a relationship.

Of course you want a partner you find physically attractive, but fancying someone isn't enough. You also have to find someone who you're going to want to spend the rest of your life with. That's a long time! When you consider the stresses and strains that come with children, jobs, and the ups and downs that are an inevitable part of being on this planet – you need the right person by your side.

Your interests and values should be in common too. You can't afford to get to that point where you've had kids and realise, in all honesty, that you and that other human being want and value completely different things. As always, it begins with being honest with yourself. When you're brutally honest with yourself, it gives you the space to be brutally honest with others.

Ask yourself what sort of energy that person is giving off. Are they positive or negative? Do they seem like somebody who's hiding something? Be curious about them. Ask questions of them. Challenge them. Find out what makes them tick and what's important to them. Work out what the other person's priorities are and respect them.

The last thing you should be looking for is someone who agrees with everything you say. The day my wife just accepts my decisions rather than challenges them is the day

I know something's wrong. It's *good* that she gives me shit. Embrace the different perspectives they offer. You want to have lots of moments where you end up saying, 'Oh, I didn't know that' or, 'Yes, of course, I hadn't thought of it like that.' When you have a great connection with somebody, you're both secure in the relationship. You can give and take criticism without the situation spiralling into a nasty row.

One thing to remember is that forming a connection with another human being isn't a one-off event. It's not a question of buying your ticket and never having to lift a finger ever again. Your partner will change over the months and years, just as you will. So don't make the mistake of assuming that they're going to keep on being the same person that you first met.

Nobody's perfect, and you'll go through bad moments and rough patches, but you should always be looking for progression in your relationships. What can you work on? What can you improve? It's one of the things that keeps you interested and engaged – and it gives you a shared project. It keeps that connection strong.

EVERYONE HAS A STORY TO TELL, IT'S UP TO YOU TO HELP THEM FIND IT

If you want to make an impression, if you want to get on in life, you have to be able to forge connections with other people. Finding common ground is the best place to start. So go out, talk to people, get to know them. I don't mean you should be out there trying to dominate conversations to the point that nobody else can get a word in edgeways. You don't want to be that pissed, bigmouthed twat, so don't butt into conversations just for the sake of having something to say.

And whatever you do, stay the fuck away from small talk. I despise small talk. I just don't have time for it. It sucks away precious minutes that I could be spending with my wife and children, and makes me feel as if I'm wasting my life. I hate having to engage in meaningless chats about the weather or holidays or football games that nobody actually cares much about. The only thing you'll ever get from irrelevant chat is irrelevant information. You're doing it to fill space and be polite, not because you're genuinely interested in the other people you're talking to.

But if you take the time and effort to wait and listen and observe you'll find an opportunity to make a connection. There will always be one thing that enables two people to relate to each other. Everyone has a story, everyone has something interesting to say. Remember that just one word or phrase can inspire another person. People inspire me every single day. I don't look to celebrities – what I'm interested in are the life experiences of ordinary people. The messages and stories I receive are incredible fuel for me. And the men and women who send me them often don't realise the impact they have. They think that because I don't reply to them that I haven't bothered to read them. That's not true at all. I might not have time to compose the response that I know they deserve, but I try to absorb every fragment of what people want to share with me.

You'll probably not know before you walk into a room who it is you'll be able to reach, but there will be somebody. And other people will want to learn from you.

I KNOW IT'S not possible to click a switch and instantly become a confident, happy, outgoing person. I know that for many people the mere *idea* of approaching someone else and starting a conversation is the stuff of nightmares, although you can get better and more capable at this sort of thing; see Chapter 2 on building confidence.

I can sense when people are shy. So I love it when I can see somebody has made the effort to overcome that in order to try to conduct a meaningful conversation with me. I'd prefer to talk to them than to a lad who's just interested in the sound of his own voice.

I'll open up the conversation as much as I can, give the person I'm talking to cues, and let them have the time and space in which to express themselves. I do the same whenever I go into somebody else's house, and I'll always try to get a conversation out of a child. You walk in and instantly they're running to hide behind their mum or dad's legs. Their parents will often say something like, 'My boy never talks to anybody.' Right, I always think, let's see if I can change that. I'm the same with adults; I see it as a challenge.

Not long ago I went round to my business partner's home. I'd never met his boy before, and he warned me that he was really antisocial. He even apologised in advance. But as far as I'm concerned there's no such thing as an antisocial child. The second I walked in he disappeared behind his mum. I noticed two things. First, he was quite nervous. And second, he was gripping a Mickey Mouse pen tightly.

I got down on my haunches. 'Hello, little man. I've got a son, same age as you. He's a little bit smaller than you, though. You're a big boy. Are you strong?' That didn't do much. He wouldn't respond and if anything tried to get even further behind his mum's legs. So I carried on. 'Oh, you've got a Minnie Mouse pen.'

That got his attention. He looked from the pen, to me, and back again. 'No, it's *Mickey* Mouse.'

'Nooooo, that's not Mickey Mouse. That's Minnie Mouse. Can I have a look?'

I stayed where I was, and he walked over to give me the pen.

'Oh yes! You're right. It *is* Mickey Mouse. Why did I think it was Minnie? Why was I being so silly? They *do* look the same, I guess –'

He interrupted me. 'No, they don't.' Then a huge flood of words started pouring out of his mouth as he patiently explained all the various ways in which they were different.

'Do you have any other pens? Could I have a look?'

He glanced up at his mum to check it was OK, then scurried off, before coming back with a mountain of pens. We talked about where he bought them, how much they cost, what different things he used them for. By the end I could barely get him to stop.

Children aren't that different from adults, and the same principles apply when it comes to trying to locate common ground. That person you're trying to talk to might not be carrying a Mickey Mouse pen, but if you're willing to watch and listen and make the effort, you'll soon find some shared interest, some point of connection, that will help unlock a meaningful conversation.

LESSONS

Good relationships are built on strong connections. Don't be swayed by superficial qualities. Make sure that you share similar values and priorities. Lust is not enough!

Every relationship is a shared project. The true value of that bond isn't in how good it is in the first month, it's how it looks after five, then ten years.

Energy never lies. We're all constantly giving off energy that tells other people who we really are. No matter what we *say* about ourselves, the energy we throw out will always tell the truth.

Life is too short for small talk. Avoid bullshit conversation. Talk about things that you actually care about.

Find common ground. Common ground is the bridge that allows human beings to make meaningful connections. Work out what's important to other people, then engage with them using what you've learned.

CHAPTER 11

CONTROL YOUR EMOTIONS, DON'T LET THEM CONTROL YOU

Acknowledge your feelings, understand them and make them work for you.

I'VE BEEN TOLD that I'm emotionless because I don't react in the way people expect me to when I'm under pressure or confronted by a tragedy. But somebody who's emotionless has cut themselves off from their feelings. In fact, they're afraid of those feelings. They're scared to expose them, because they know that they cannot control them.

That's not me. I'm incredibly connected to my emotions. I've exposed them time and time again, which means that I can control them.

I'm not fearless. Far from it. But I get excited when I feel fear. It's an emotion I've made work for me. I exposed it so many times on the battlefield, and then again and again in so many other contexts, that I am totally familiar with it. I'm in control of it.

That control is why, when we used to storm compounds, I could switch effortlessly from the cold fury needed to fire rounds into an insurgent's chest, to the empathy required to calm a room full of terrified women and children. It's why I can look at an emotion, decide it's no good for the particular situation I'm facing, and park it up.

So I'm not emotionless. What I am, however, is emotionally intelligent.

Emotional intelligence is understanding any given emotion for what it is, and then making that emotion work for you. The majority of people spend their whole time on the planet battling against themselves. They see their moods and behaviour as impenetrable mysteries and have never invested time in understanding themselves. This means that they're continually surprised when they lose their temper or aren't able to find motivation.

These people aren't willing to commit to the process of understanding what the emotion is, whether it's anger, pain, suffering, sadness or fear. That's a mistake, because the moment that emotion isn't working *for* you it's going to start working *against* you. You should be looking to control your emotions, not let your emotions control you.

If you're not willing to find out how you function, how are you going to be able to identify what you need to work on? A life lived on autopilot is no kind of life at all. There's no growth, no challenge. More than that, when people don't do that work of exposing their emotions, they're vulnerable. A new emotion hits them and they don't know how to react. They run away or break down.

We're all human, which means we all have weaknesses and insecurities. If you take the time to identify them, you can deal with them. If you try to ignore your demons, they'll end up running the show behind the scenes.

I've seen intelligent, level-headed soldiers lose their heads on the battlefield. They come running past you, behaving in a way that shocks you. You look into their eyes and there's nothing there, so you can only ask: 'Wow, where the *hell* did that come from?' They're people that haven't confronted the emotions inside them; instead they've brushed them off or pretended that they don't exist. And now these emotions have surged up and taken control.

For me, this would be like going through life with one arm tied behind your back. If you're locking an emotion off, you're restricting who you could become and what you can achieve.

Take anger. It's a fucking important emotion. If you can't control it, anger can be a liability. If you can control it, you can use it as fuel to drive you on further than you ever thought possible. So if you just block it off, you're denying yourself 20, maybe 30 per cent of your potential.

The first thing to remember is that your emotions are you. There's no gap between you and your anger. That anger is as much a part of you as your blue eyes. Everyone's emotions are completely different. Your emotions are as individual to you as your facial features, or the sound of your voice. Only you can know your emotions fully, and only you can control them. Nobody else can do that work for you.

Your task is to reach that point where you know your emotions intimately. I know it takes courage and I appreciate that it can be uncomfortable, sometimes unpleasant. But it's work that will repay the effort a million times over. People who are familiar with and in control of their emotions are far closer to operating at their optimal level than those who aren't. Your decisions will be better, you'll be better able to relate to others, you'll cope better in stressful situations.

TAKE THE LAYERS OFF

The most courageous thing you can do in life is to expose your emotions. I realise now how courageous it was to have sat down on my bed and berated myself for my inability to get through that door. I was confronting my fears. Even now, I'm harder on myself than any recruit that has ever been on *SAS: Who Dares Wins*. And I do that every single day.

You can't acquire this type of information by sitting alone in a quiet, dark room. It's life that teaches you. So go out there, expose yourself to different situations, then repeat the process, over and over again. You might get things wrong, you might get them right. It doesn't matter. Fuck what other people think of you. You're learning about yourself. Why limit your ability to do that just because some other prick has started sniggering.

When you feel something, don't just let it float away: grab it, study it. If you fly into a temper, don't pretend that it hasn't happened. Make a note to yourself of what triggered you or what the signs of that anger growing in you were. What *exactly* were you feeling in the seconds immediately before you completely lost your shit?

I won't pretend this an easy process. It involves pain. So I completely understand how people might experience, say, fear once and decide that they don't ever want to go anywhere near it again. They wrap themselves in cotton wool, terrified of their vulnerability. They will never challenge themselves and because of that they'll be forever limited.

Some people commit to exposing their emotions, but they go about it in the wrong way – often by trying to bite off too much of the emotion at once. So, for instance, they decide that the best way to conquer their fear of heights is to chuck themselves off a massive bridge attached to the end of a bungee cord. At best they'll get a huge surge of adrenaline that gives them the fuel to push themselves over the edge. More likely they'll approach it and become so gripped by the terror of vertigo that they get paralysed and go back home with their tail between their legs. Either way, the result is effectively the same. They've attempted to take too big a bite, realised they are not going to be able to swallow it and then completely changed their minds. Anything they might have learned about themselves or their emotions has been discarded. All they have left is the fear that they started with.

Build up gradually. If you want to address your fear of heights walk halfway up a fucking steepish hill. Stay there for a moment, *feel* that vertigo, *feel* that fear. Then go straight back down. The emotion is still there, but you've taken a layer off it. Next time you approach the hill, you'll know that you've already experienced some of that emotion. You've felt it and survived. Then it's time to take another layer off. You might go a bit higher. You repeat that process. Little by little you'll be taking positive steps forward. Don't feel any pressure to rush. It might take two or three attempts; it might take two or three weeks; it might take two or three years. That's fine. You've got time on your side.

This is a process you can carry on for the rest of your life with so many other emotions.

BREAK IT DOWN

After each mission came the official debrief, in which we'd analyse in forensic detail what had happened – what had gone well, what had gone wrong; how closely we'd been able to follow and execute the original plan; how we'd responded to the curveballs that the situation threw at us.

Once this was over and we'd all trooped off to our various corners of the base, I'd conduct the same exercise but I'd be focused only on myself. I'd break everything down and think not just about what I'd done, but how I'd felt. Most of the time I was happy, because although I wouldn't have been able to articulate it quite so clearly then, deep down I knew that I was connected to myself and as a result was more often than not making the right decision for the right reasons. I'd think about that guy where I *didn't* pull the trigger, where in the heat of combat I could have put ten rounds into his skull, ripped his teeth out and worn them as a necklace, but instead lowered my rifle.

When it comes to your own emotions, it's so crucial to break what you're feeling down. Now when an emotion presents itself, my first question is: what am I feeling? That's followed by: why am I feeling like this?

If you're angry, you need to ask yourself why. Be honest about the situation you're in. When you're driving your kids to school and some twat cuts you up just as you're trying to park, you'll probably feel a surge a rage. Instead of leaping out of your car and getting in the other driver's face, take a moment to acknowledge what you're feeling and why. Once you've named something, you've started to take control over it. If you don't acknowledge and name that feeling, it's going to whirl out of control and start working against you. The more you expose your emotions to the jagged edges of life, the more layers you're going to take off. The more layers you take off, the more you'll understand that emotion.

Acknowledge the emotion. Only then is it time to decide whether to take an action. Ask yourself whether what you're about to do is going to result in a positive or a negative. If you're in the grip of road rage and you get out of the car to confront the other driver, it's likely to result in a fight. You start off screaming, 'Fucking wanker, pull over,' you end up doing something you regret or pushing that other guy into doing something *he regrets*. Either way, it's a very fucking sub-par outcome.

Once you've framed what you're doing and why, that will inform everything. It will affect both your conscious and your instinctive reactions. It will mean that you can take that negative emotion and flip it into a positive.

Let's take another situation. Say I'm climbing up a mountain and I'm still 100 metres from the summit. My feet are blistered, my hands cut to shreds, then I start to get angry with myself. Why am I feeling rage? Because I'm in a shit state. Is there a positive to actioning my anger? Yes, I can use it to drive me on to my goal. The next few minutes are fucking dreadful, but it's that aggression that helps me endure them. I had a positive motivator.

That's what I used to help me get through doors when I was in the SBS. If I stayed put, I'd fucking die. My positive motivator was staying alive.

If you haven't exposed that emotion before, when fear or anger present themselves, you won't recognise it for what it is. You won't break that feeling down, you don't take that minute to pause and you'll end up overwhelmed. So if you're angry, you'll find yourself flying off the handle.

DON'T BE A LEAKY VESSEL

The idea that you should let your emotions out whenever you want is bullshit. You need to control your emotions because you need to control yourself. You have a responsibility to people other than yourself. If I'm feeling angry, is it acceptable for me to go around punching people in the face? Clearly not. It's the same with sadness.

If you're a fucking leaky vessel, if you're not in charge of your emotions, people will take advantage of you. They'll abuse and manipulate your emotions. I used to think it was OK to just let your anger go free when you were provoked. If five or six years ago somebody had told me that being a man would involve ignoring the fucker who bashed into you deliberately rather than smashing his face into mince, I'd have laughed.

But the penny has dropped now. It might be satisfying for about thirty seconds to embrace that red mist. But every time I've done it I've either ended up in a police cell or in prison with bruised knuckles. Nothing positive ever came from letting my anger go free, and when I did the consequences could have destroyed my family. Now I understand that being a man is actually about knowing yourself, about having the emotional intelligence to make the right decision in a split second. That's so much more important than 'saving face'. You're not proving anything, you're not taking responsibility. And you're not going anywhere.

But as important as it is to control your emotions, you should never make the mistake of repressing them. You must give them an outlet, otherwise they'll make themselves known in uncomfortable ways further down the line, or they'll stay unexamined inside you causing trouble, like a disruptive, malevolent presence. Emotional dumps are so crucial to resetting your emotional equilibrium. When I was out kicking doors down or caught up in firefights, it was clearly the wrong time to let all my emotions spill out. I would wait until later, when I was back at base. That's when I might let myself shed a tear. A few years later, when I watched my mum die in hospital, I had to keep strong for her and for everybody else gathered around her bed. But I wept the whole way home. It's not weak to need that release – it's an essential part of your emotional hygiene. You just have to choose your moments.

NEVER STOP TAKING THE LAYERS OFF

The ability to control your emotions is like any other skill. You've got to practise it. In fact, you should make it a life-long project. With every year that goes by you should be looking to become stronger, wiser and more knowledgeable. It's a virtuous circle. When you start to understand your emotions, you'll have a better understanding of yourself. When you have a better understand of yourself, you'll know what you're capable of. And when you know what you're capable of, your confidence will grow.

The moment you stop that process, you stop learning and growing as an individual. A lot of people reach a certain stage in life and their attitude becomes, 'Oh, been there, done that.' They stop challenging themselves, and they end up wasting years and years of their lives. Whatever emotional intelligence they've acquired shrivels, like muscles that atrophy because they're not being exercised. But my attitude is: why wouldn't you want to keep evolving?

That's why even after I left the military I continued to put myself in extreme situations that engendered extreme emotions. That's why I climbed Mount Everest during a storm. That's why I starved myself in the blazing heat of the Pacific Ocean. I never want to stop taking those layers off.

LESSONS

You can learn to control your emotions. If you don't make that effort, they will end up controlling you.

Your emotional make-up is unique to you. Only you can do the work of becoming intimately familiar with your emotions. Break what you're feeling down. What is it? Why is it happening now? Keep asking questions until you know those feelings inside out.

Expose your emotions before they expose you. You have to go out and expose your emotions to the world. Make sure you know what anger or fear *feels* like.

Letting go isn't always good. You should never repress your emotions, but nor should you let them run riot. Children scream and shout when they don't get what they want, children smash shit when they're angry. Adults don't.

Never stop taking those layers off. The moment you get complacent about your emotions is the moment you will start to lose control over them.

CHAPTER 12

HARD TIMES DON'T LAST, HARD MEN DO

How to build resilience.

MY MUM DIED during the first frightening weeks of the Covid lockdown in March 2020.

She had been diagnosed with cancer at the end of 2019, and for a while there was talk of a course of chemotherapy and a vaguely optimistic prognosis. If the chemo worked, it might give her another year, maybe even two. In the end, she only had three months left.

I was busy with work, and in and out of the country. Messages between me and my sister, who lived with Mum in Paignton, got a bit disjointed, as they often do when you're suddenly struggling with an event of this magnitude. And then the pandemic scrambled things even more. If I'd known how little time was left, I'd have spent more precious time with her. Hindsight can be the cruellest thing. I only managed a day alongside her after finding out she was ill, and then the lockdown came into force. It was a horrible, horrible time.

By the end of March her condition started to deteriorate quite rapidly. She went into hospital, supposedly just on a temporary basis, but she stayed there. By the time I was able to come to see her again she'd already had a stroke, which left her able to communicate only through faint hand squeezes.

I found her lying in bed, looking small and impossibly frail in the bright hospital light. Wires ran in and out of her body, attached to a battery of machines. I felt my heart start to break. Mum was a proud, dignified woman. She would never have wanted for any of us to see her in that state.

She had stage 4 cancer, the sickness having spread through her body so quickly that they were unable even to identify the primary cancer. It was now in her lungs and her thyroid – her body was failing her. My mum was plainly nearing the end of her life. It was touch and go whether she'd even make it through the night. She was weak and broken, suffering from almost unimaginable pain, and the fact that she could no longer communicate properly with us had left her agitated and frantic.

I stepped outside the ward for a couple of minutes to talk to my sister. She had been amazing for so long. During the lonely, tough weeks after Mum had first fallen sick, my sister had taken so much pressure and responsibility on her shoulders. So much, I think, that she'd reached the point where it all began to feel overwhelming.

'I can't do it,' she said, tears pouring down her cheeks. 'My heart feels as if it's about to break. I can't make any decisions. Suddenly I don't know what she wants or needs. I knew this moment would come, but it's all too much.'

In my old life I'd looked after the dead bodies of my brothers-in-arms. As horrible as things were in this quiet, still, overpoweringly warm hospital ward, I realised those experiences ensured that I had the composure needed to take charge of the situation. It didn't mean that seeing Mum like this didn't hurt, but it did mean I was psychologically prepared. My emotions weren't running out of control and I could look at things with a clear head. If there was nothing that could be done to save our mother, we could at least make sure that her last hours with us were as painless as possible.

'Don't worry,' I told my sister, 'I've got this'

I found the nurse. 'Mum's in a real bad way,' I told her. 'She's suffering, she's in pain, so much pain. She's got secondaries in her lungs and her thyroid. Her cancer's everywhere. We need to help her.'

'It's begun already,' she said. 'The stroke was a sign of her body shutting down. We can't stop this happening.'

'I know, but can we help make it as easy as we can for her? I can't imagine the discomfort she must be in.'

The nurse nodded and gestured for me to follow her as she searched for the doctor. We agreed to increase the level of pain relief we'd give her.

We went back to Mum's bedside. I took her hand. 'The nurses are coming, Mum. You haven't got long left, and they're going to help you feel better. I'm going to be right by your side all the way.'

I talked to her for a bit longer, and then we waited. I could feel that for the first time in hours she was completely relaxed. I sat there with her as her finger stroked the top of my hand. I'd been here before with comrades. I knew what she was feeling, I knew what she was going through.

A little while after the morphine went in her body settled down. Her breathing changed, grew slower. The panic that had earlier gripped her body was now replaced by a kind of serenity.

Twelve more hours elapsed until she finally passed. We all sat in that room together, saying very little, just watching her chest rise and fall. Doctors and nurses walked softly past us, occasionally coming to check in low voices if we needed anything. The only other sounds were the intermittent bleeps of the machines beside my mum's bed.

Then, slowly, very slowly, without any sort of ceremony, she slipped away. The cancer had finally taken her. Within half an hour we packed up all her belongings. I managed to stay strong all the way to her last breath, and it was only once I set out on the drive across country to my home that I started to cry.

*   *   *

IN THE DAYS that followed I missed her sharply. It was a feeling of loss I hadn't experienced for years. Even if we might have had our differences, I'd never fallen out with my mum, although our busy lives meant that we didn't see that much of each other. I always knew that she loved me, and I loved her.

Mum's death was the hardest challenge I've ever had to face. In fact it was probably the worst thing that has happened to me since my memories began. It was also deeply personal. So it's not something I've talked about much in public, and it's not been plastered all over my social media. Lots of people kept on saying how well I was dealing with it, and some concluded that I don't feel emotion like everybody else does. I can assure you, I do. Seeing my mum take her last breaths was heartbreaking. She'd asked for me because she knew I'd be there for her, as I always had been. And when it came to it, I was able to call on the emotions I needed to smooth her last hours on the planet.

In some ways, much of my life was a preparation for the moments I spent beside my mum's hospital bed. The resilience I was able to show was the positive result of the suffering I've been through.

Losing my dad and then my nan when I was still so young was fucking awful. But one of the consequences was that later, when I lost friends in combat, I was prepared; these situations weren't as traumatic for me as they were for some of the other lads. My time in the regular armed forces means that I can see a dead body and remain calm when everybody else might be losing their shit, because I've been on the battlefield and seen hundreds of dead bodies. I've taken life. I've saved life. That, in turn, was preparation for the unrelenting pressure of the Special Forces, which was as much a test of mental resilience as it was physical strength. Every day I was walking that line that separates the bright world of the living from the dark void we'll all enter one day. You have to live with your decisions. You have to live with what you've seen and done. You have to live with what you take back from the battlefield.

In the years that I worked in Africa and South America I saw gangs, corruption, gratuitous violence – the worst of humanity. It was horrible at the time, but I've come to see it as a blessing. All of that was a well of experience that I found I could draw on. It taught me that experiencing hardship and suffering shows you what you're really made of. You discover your inner grit, your inner strength, your inner steel. It turns out that whatever doesn't kill you really does make you stronger.

THAT'S LIFE, SON

In the course of your time on this planet you'll experience loss, anger and sadness. It's horrible, but nobody's spared that pain.

Many of us have a tendency to dwell on joy, happiness, success and positivity, but you can't live in that world alone. You can't pretend the other things aren't out there. The world *can* be cruel and robust. Being alive *can* hurt. It's a massive cliché, but sometimes bad things do happen. There are times when the only response to a problem your child brings you is: 'But that's life, son.'

Say one of my boys comes to me crying because another kid has accidentally kicked a ball into his face and then laughed afterwards. I can see it's upsetting and a bit humiliating, but it's just one of those things that happens.

First off I'd ask him, 'If you'd done the same, kicked a ball into his face, do you think you'd let out a little snigger?'

'Yes.'

'Because it's funny, isn't it? Quite funny, anyway. And it's an accident. He wasn't doing it maliciously or on purpose. These things happen.'

So an important part of developing resilience is acknowledging the dark elements that are an unavoidable part of being human. We need to understand that bad things will happen to us, and that we'll have to find ways of coping when they do. We also need to familiarise ourselves with our emotional make-up and the demons that we all have inside us. This is crucial, because they are the things that will determine how we respond when it all kicks off. I fought with some soldiers who went to war without ever taking the time to understand what lived inside them. I'm not sure they even knew that their demons existed. But when they were put under extreme stress the demons emerged, and these soldiers ended up doing things that they later found very hard to live with.

THE KINDNESS TRAP

Just like everything else I've discussed so far in this book, resilience isn't something you can simply will into existence – you have to work at building it. Like confidence and emotional control, resilience is the product of experience. You gain resilience by going through tough times and coming out the other side. Each time you're faced with struggle or discomfort you'll learn a little bit more about yourself, you'll grow a little more.

That's why parents have such an incredibly important role in the process of their children acquiring resilience. The earlier we begin to acquire an inner fortitude, the better we will be at coping with stuff further down the line.

Unfortunately, we're a nation of lazy fathers and mothers. Instead of helping our children grow and mature and learn, we stick them in front of iPads. I get so mad when I go to restaurants and see kids scrolling through their phones when they should be eating and talking.

And so many of us aren't entirely truthful with our children. Rather than talking honestly about the world, we try to shelter them from it with white lies. Sugarcoating can seem to work, superficially at least. Years can go by without this tiptoeing around the hard facts of life causing any difficulty, and then suddenly something dramatic happens or the kid just goes out unprotected into the big wide world, and they find themselves overwhelmed. It's too much for them to handle.

I also cannot bear those parents who complain when their kid gets told off at school.

'It's unfair, why are they picking on her?'

'It's probably because your girl is a little shit.'

'No, no, that's not my girl.'

'Well, they haven't done their homework.'

'Yeah, it's *ridiculous* how much they get.'

Dude, you're doing your child no favours at all. You don't understand what life is all about. Children need to learn what it's like to be told off. There are other parents who shit themselves when they see their kid crying because her team has lost a football match. Good, I think. They *should* be crying. I'd be crying too if I was in the same position. But guess what, you suck it up and you crack on. I want my kids to know what it's like to come last. You gain so much from exposing that emotion, taking the layers.

What you should be doing is helping your kids establish that small store of emotional resilience that they can draw on when something far bigger and badder comes full pelt at them further down the line.

Some people get this. I was speaking with a guy the other day who'd bought a dog for his family. There were loads of reasons for doing so, he said. But one of the principal motivations for him was knowing that the dog would live happily alongside his kids for a decade or so, and then would come to the end of his natural lifespan. He wanted his children to understand what that emotion was. He wanted them to feel loss that they could manage so that then when bigger, more wrenching losses came, they'd be primed.

This isn't to say that I don't understand how hard it is to be an active part in this process. It's not just the effort involved, it's also the need to overcome the desire that exists in all of us to wrap our children in cotton wool to protect them from all of the world's sharp edges. I'm as guilty of succumbing to that temptation as anybody else.

There are days when I watch them scamper up ladders to their treehouses and there's part of me that wants to race over, hold their hands steady so they don't fall, or add a fucking handrail so that all possible risk is removed. I have to tell myself, *Ant, get a grip*.

I do, however, have a stronger stomach than Emilie. My four-year-old drives around our garden in a go-kart built for a thirteen-year-old. As he whizzes about at 15 mph doing laps, Emilie can barely look. 'Oh my life, what are you letting him *do*? I'm getting chest pains.' But he's in a crash helmet, he's strapped in securely. The worst thing that could happen is that he'll crash into the fence and break a bit of the wood. He won't be hurt, but he'll learn a lesson.

And, of course, that's exactly what he did do. He smashed into that fence, we rushed over and there he was, looking around. A bit surprised, but absolutely fine. Now when he goes round those corners he's not going to make the mistake of accelerating when he should brake. I'd told him that's what he'd needed to do, but of course he hadn't listened. He had to actually have that little smash-up to learn the lesson. He's also taken a layer off his fear.

That's an amazing advantage to give your children. And yet I know there are so many people out there that will read this and just think that I'm a fucking irresponsible, reckless parent who's too willing to shove their kids into dangerous situations. I guess that's just the society we live in now. Parents are worried about following their instincts, doing what they know is right, because they're worried about what others will think.

Fuck them. I've *seen* what works for my kids. And, furthermore, what works for my kids will work for you too. The principles are exactly the same. Life will send challenges your way, but why wait? Why not try to ensure that when something really does come along and kicks you in the teeth, you're ready to deal with it. Seek out those challenges yourself. Do things that make you uncomfortable. Nobody ever built resilience by staying in bed.

THE MOST POWERFUL TOOL
ON THE PLANET

It's worth remembering that although resilience might seem like a fairly modern concept, what lies beneath it is as ancient as we are. People claim to like, even need, comfort. But we weren't designed to be comfortable. So much of life these days is constructed to be as easy and frictionless as possible. There are apps that do all of our navigating and remembering for us, rules that tell us what we can and can't do, where we can and can't go.

It goes against the grain of our being to be stuck in that mode of existence. That's not who we are as a species. Mankind has always thrived on danger and excitement, on pushing itself beyond boundaries. That's us at our best. We used to spend our energy trying to put people on the moon; now mankind's main aim seems to be seeing how much of its existence it can conduct without ever having to leave the couch.

At times it feels to me as if we're being forced to turn off the most powerful tool on the planet: the human brain. We're being asked to leave it dormant. To avoid falling into this trap I put myself in horrendous situations where I have to fight against myself. If I'm in a context that's unfamiliar to me, that I know nothing about, it makes me work, it pushes me to think in ways I wouldn't normally, it pushes me into uncomfortable places. Good, that's what's going to make me stronger. If I'd have gone up Mount Everest on a nice sunny day, I'd have gained nothing from that experience.

TAKE THE REINS

For me, being resilient is not just about being able to cope with an adverse situation, it's about being able to act within it. It's a dynamic not a passive quality.

When a difficult situation is forced upon you, you're faced with two choices: you can either crack or cope. And if you can cope, then you might find you can thrive. You can make it work for you. These are the situations that make you realise what you're capable of.

People will say about my mum's death, 'Ant, you were so fucking brave.' I don't agree. And yet there I was. As I saw it, I had two choices: I could have collapsed in a heap weeping, in the process destroying myself and my family, or I could have stepped up to the mark, used my life experience – yep, I'll draw on that emotion, I'll remember how a particular moment felt.

When you think about it, it's not a difficult choice.

What can seem difficult is the prospect of controlling or even understanding those sorts of moments, but I'd like you to realise that you can completely reframe your approach to them. And the key to success in tackling an adverse situation is to adopt a positive mindset. Lean into the problem, don't just sit there waiting for another bucket of shit to be poured over your head.

The first thing I do is to strip everything back, see the situation for what it is, then work out what I can do to wrest back control. I want to live a life full of courageous decisions that I step into. I want to force a decision on the world rather than have the world forcing a decision on me. Whenever I can, I try to get moving. I want to restore my sense of agency and momentum.

Don't let yourself get bogged down by the fear of making a bad decision. It's far worse to be so paralysed that you make no decision at all. I'll always stand by somebody who makes a decision and fucks up. The military is geared to helping you make good, quick decisions. Combat is not an environment that's particularly friendly to people who dither. You haven't got time *not* to decide. If you fuck about it's going to cost lives. *You* might not have made your mind up, but you can bet your fucking life that the enemy will have.

When you postpone those hard decisions you're really just prolonging the agony. You can't rely on the crisis just sorting itself out because you haven't the guts to do something. Life doesn't work like that. Once a problem presents itself, you have to find a solution. Making decisions, even the wrong ones, gets you closer to that solution.

If you adopt a leadership mentality in those situations you'll find them easier. Being a leader demands that you take responsibility, make decisions and think of others before you consider yourself.

I couldn't stop my mum from dying, but I could try to do as much as possible to ease her pain as she slipped away. In order to make that momentous decision, I had to put some of my emotions to one side. My energy and focus had to be on her suffering, not on how I felt.

It's so tempting to let yourself be overwhelmed by how you feel. It's much better to focus your mind on what you can *do*. The more control you can exert over a situation, the better chance you have of understanding and processing what you're experiencing, and the more likely you are to find a solution.

Taking control of a situation isn't a question of running around barking orders. Often that noisy behaviour is a sign of precisely the opposite. What it means is that you have taken the effort to work out what's happening and what actions you need to take in response. It means that you understand what emotions you are feeling, and in doing so you are not letting them overwhelm you. Think about what's in front of you. Strip away all the distractions until you can make sense of it. It's as if it's sitting there in the palm of my hand. Everyone can do that. I'll never tire of saying this: if you don't make the situation work for you, then it's going to work against you.

WE'RE ALMOST ALWAYS STRONGER THAN WE THINK

Whenever you're in the middle of a particularly difficult moment, try to take a few seconds to remind yourself of all the occasions in your past when you've got through tough times. I did that when I was trying to ease my mum's last moments. I thought about what I'd seen and done in Afghanistan. I didn't sugarcoat it and pretend those experiences had been pleasant, but I did think about the fact that I'd survived them. *They hadn't broken me then, so why would I fall to pieces now?* We're almost always stronger than we think.

LESSONS

Bad things will happen. There is pain and misery in the world. Sometimes life gets hard. Anybody who pretends different is setting themselves up for an almighty fucking fall.

Don't get caught in the kindness trap. The sooner your kids get exposed to the world's rough edges, the better they'll be able to deal with them.

Nobody ever got resilient by staying in their bedroom. Put yourself in tricky situations, make yourself uncomfortable, give yourself experience of being under pressure. Every small challenge you survive is the most amazing practice for that moment when a really big challenge descends upon you.

When things go wrong, adopt a leadership mentality. Do what you can to seize control of the situation. Taking the initiative is the first step towards solving the problem.

A bad decision is better than no decision. Doing nothing helps nobody, but every wrong answer brings you closer to the right one.

You're already resilient. Never underestimate yourself. You've survived so much shit in life and you're still standing. Use the resilience you already possess as a foundation, and keep on building on it.

CHAPTER 13

YOU CAN BREAK THROUGH THE PAIN BARRIER

How to use your mind to help your body smash through its limits.

Winter Hills, Brecon Beacons, January 2008

You wake up in the morning full of a mix of dread and excitement. The end of this phase of Selection is close, so unbelievably close, and yet you know you still have to go through sixty kilometres of hell. The 'Long Drag', as the Special Forces call it, is a battle against steep Welsh mountains and vicious Welsh weather. You're carrying seventy pounds on your back, with your weapon in your arms and the accumulated aches, pains and exhaustion of the last weeks of Selection in your limbs.

We'd all been through so much already. Selection is designed to be painful. It's supposed to be so difficult that only a tiny percentage of candidates pass. They make it hard because the missions the SBS are sent on are hard, full of physical and mental pain. Killing people hurts. They had to be absolutely fucking *certain* that if we found ourselves in the middle of any mission, any environment, any catastrophe, we'd have the mental and physical wherewithal to cope.

We'd had a month of being thrashed in the Brecon Beacons, and there had already been a week and a half of timed marches. Everything we did was a test, designed to push us to our utter limits, every task another way of asking the same question, again and again. Do you possess that sheer, bloody-minded determination to push on through, whatever the conditions, no matter how fucked you are in body and mind? Two hundred and twenty men had started my course. That number had been whittled down day after day, as lads either chucked it in or were hauled off by one of the instructors. I knew that maybe forty at most would make it through to the jungle. I was determined to be one of them.

I remember just standing there in the few peaceful seconds before the ordeal began. It wasn't just a test of raw physical endurance; we had to do all the navigation ourselves – the old-fashioned way with map and compass. And all the time, there was the pressure of having to complete the course in under twenty hours. Neither our bodies nor our minds would have a moment's rest. It hadn't been raining when I'd first opened my eyes. It was now. The water was coming down hard and fast, whipped by an angry wind that billowed around as if it had a grudge against us. I knew that the rain would be soaking remorselessly into the soft Welsh soil. There would be churning mud that sucked and gripped at my boots. Every footstep today would be treacherous, every stone slippery.

I looked up at the looming mass of the Brecon Beacons. The scale of the task was almost too big to digest, the downpour now so heavy that my vision had become blurry. It was hard sometimes to make out details on the map as water streamed across its surface and pooled in its folds.

I wiped my eyes, made sure I was heading in the right direction, then took a decisive step forwards. Time to go.

MY SHINS WERE already aching, my calves already burning, and everything in my body seemed to be screaming at me at once. I had expected this. What I hadn't planned for was that all of this pain would kick in after only thirty minutes. I struggled to process the idea that I still had over nineteen hours to go. It didn't seem possible that so little time had elapsed, yet I was already so uncomfortable.

Fifteen minutes later everything was different. I began to feel warmed up, my muscles were flexing, my blood was pumping. It was still pissing down, I was still having to wipe freezing rain out of my eyes every few seconds and every step was a battle with viscous red mud – but things were good. *Fuck me*, I thought, *I think I can actually do this*. One hour passed, then another, I was still in a good place ... then the pendulum swung again. Hard. As the three-hour mark approached I realised how fatigued I really was. Despite being in an environment that appeared to be 90 per cent water, I was dehydrated. My throat was dry and I could feel an uncomfortable pulse behind my temples. I knew that the sheer effort involved in struggling up and over the mountains meant I was burning far more calories than I could possibly take in. I could feel my energy ebbing away at precisely the same time as the pain inside me reached new levels. That's when the suffering really began.

After three hours a numbing pain began to spread slowly: first my legs, then up through my torso, then into my arms. My body was one whole dull fucking ache, like the discomfort that lies heavily in your limbs when you have a bad attack of flu, except magnified by a thousand. Every atom in my body was vibrating with pain – there was nothing sharp or stabbing, it was a slow, relentless accumulation of agony, as if my organs and limbs were beginning the process of shutting down. It was pain that left me fighting with myself. Because that's the thing with pain. It's not just something that happens in your body.

One voice in my head was saying, *I can't go on.* Another was saying, *Just put one foot in front of the other.*

I'd been told that the Long Drag was as much a test of your mental fortitude as your physical strength. Now I learned that brutal truth for myself. For one thing, there was always, always, the time pressure. You're constantly anxious. Am I going to make the next checkpoint? And up there on the mountainside I felt unbelievably alone. My only companions were my pain, fear and insecurities swirling around my mind, the needles of rain stinging my face and the pitiless wind tearing endlessly at my sodden clothes.

I've got to get through this, I've got to get through this, I've got to get through this. You can't get through this, you can't get through this, you can't get through this.

Hard as I tried to stop them, unwanted voices crowded into my mind – the voices of everyone who had ever doubted me, everyone who had ever told me I wasn't good enough, that I didn't have what it took, that I'd been presumptuous to even *consider* Selection. Their faces swam in and out of view, as real to me as the lancing rain and the brutal hills of the Brecon Beacons. It was as if the pain had opened the door to all of my demons.

Why the fuck was I doing this? What was the point of all this pain? Why not give up? I was almost pleading with myself. *Just give me one reason why I shouldn't give up.*

TO BEGIN WITH, every pain feels unprecedented. You tell yourself that not only have you never been in such agony before, you begin to persuade yourself it will never end. The idea that you might be able to pass your pain threshold, the idea that your pain threshold even exists, begins to seem ludicrous.

But that was the point, I realised. This wasn't unprecedented. I *had* been here before. The very fact that I was here, struggling through mud and rock and rain, was precisely because I'd long ago learned what it meant to cross my pain threshold. Remembering this changed everything. The pain didn't diminish. If anything, it continued to grow. But I knew now with great clarity that sometime soon it would end. All I had to do was hang on in there. All I had to do was plod on, continue putting one foot in front of the other, dragging myself closer and closer to the end.

More minutes passed. The wind blew, I felt water trickling uncomfortably down my back and into my boots, and I pushed on and on. I was stumbling more now. Pain and exhaustion had left me less sure of my footing in the freezing mud, but I pushed on. *I've got to get through this, I've got to get through this, I've got to get through this.* And then something just gave. The strange thing is that when it actually occurs, a certain amount of time passes before you notice. There's nobody banging a cymbal or congratulating you. One moment you're doing everything you can to control the pain, the next you realise that the agony has gone, that your limbs feel stronger.

Often it comes when your mind is diverted. This time it happened just as I'd reached a summit and taken out my compass to plot the next leg of my route. I looked down at the steep, jagged ridge I was about to follow, and suddenly found myself gripped by an intense euphoria. It felt like a victory: I'd fought against my pain and beaten it. I took deep breaths, savouring the release from the agony of the last hour. I knew it wouldn't last. I knew that before long I'd be heading back down into that valley of pain. But somehow that intensified the sheer pleasure of the moment.

For what seemed like the millionth time that day, I wiped water from my eyes. I took a deep swig from my canteen, shook my limbs and, still giddy with elation and relief, I strode on.

I MUST HAVE hit the pain barrier three more times before I finally reached the last checkpoint. Once every four hours. Each time I knew that it was coming, like seeing a mountain in the distance. I don't think it ever got easier. In fact, as I talked about in *First Man In*, my right ankle almost gave up the ghost, leaving me in so much pain that I effectively entered a trance state. But I knew that it was something I was going to have to face – and I knew that I could get through it.

PAIN IS A funny old thing. You can't ignore it. You *shouldn't* ignore it because it has a crucial evolutionary function. It's there as a warning sign. I know there are people who say that all you need to do is 'block out the pain'. Of course, those people are idiots who nobody should be listening to. Try telling someone whose legs have just been blown to off to block out the pain.

But if you cannot ignore pain, then you can try to understand it. And once you've understood it, you can begin to control it.

Broadly speaking there are two types of pain. The first kind is pain that happens to you. It's the kind that follows an accident or getting shot or when you're on the wrong end of a nasty tackle in a football match.

In a sense, there's nothing to worry about with this type of pain. It's easy because there isn't a choice. You're going to have to deal with it, someone will probably be offering you painkillers, so why think too much about it until you have to? But it's trickier with the second type of pain, when it's something like a marathon or a hardcore tier one mission, when you know in advance that at some point you're going to be suffering. In these instances you're committing to pain. I don't mean the sort of pain that follows a broken bone; I'm talking about the feeling that descends upon you halfway through a run and makes you feel that you simply can't go take another step forward.

You can't just block this type of pain out. What you can do, however, is learn to understand where your pain threshold lies and know that you've got the capability to push right through it. And the way to do that is to expose yourself to pain for a sustained period of time, something that for quite obvious reasons a lot of people have never done.

Once you've managed that, you'll begin to appreciate that pain can make you feel alive. It makes you aware of your body and its operations in ways you'd never experience otherwise. You are in the most literal sense possible stepping outside your comfort zone, testing your body. It's one of the most exhilarating sensations I know.

That exhilaration is the result, in part at least, of the fact that it's an amazing example of the connection between body and mind. They're intricately linked in this process, one supporting the other, and both have to step up and play a role.

THE THRESHOLD

The most important thing you need to know about pain is that you have a threshold. When you push your body hard, your brain will send signals to your body urging it to reserve its energy for emergencies. It's an inbuilt protective device. But we're capable of so much more than our body thinks. And there's a point beyond which your discomfort begins to diminish, even disappear. You might need to go to the depths of hell to find it, but the journey is so worth it.

Pain is like fear or failure. The moment you experience it, you want it to stop. Your instinct is to say, *Fuck that, let's get out of here.* It feels counterintuitive to seek it out. But just like fear or failure, if you expose yourself to it, you'll be preparing yourself for the hard fucking realities of life. If you're going to do something like run a marathon, you need to give your mind and body experience of feeling uncomfortable. So, when it comes – and it will come – it won't be a shock to you.

Think of what happens when you jump into cold water. For those first few moments all you want to do is get out straight away. That's true of most people. It's too uncomfortable and they don't feel as if they can bear it for a second longer. But if you stay there for ninety seconds, maybe two minutes, your body will become acclimatised. It'll feel numb.

You've crossed the pain threshold.

When I was a kid trying to get into the Paras I couldn't get past that pain threshold. I didn't know where it was; I'm not even sure I knew it existed. We'd go out on extremely long yomps with heavy loads on our backs and at some point the straps of my Bergen would be cutting into my shoulders, my legs would be full of burning lactic acid and I'd be in such agony that I'd end up saying, 'I can't do it, I'm going to have to back out.' And that would be that. Another failure.

Then I realised I had to do the same thing with pain as I had with my emotions. I had to expose and endure it in order to understand it. After all, it was always going to be there, so why ignore it? Why pretend it didn't exist? I had to become at ease with pain. I pushed on and pushed on.

For a while the pain was still too much. I'd try to stay in it for as long as I could but eventually I'd have to say to myself, *Fuck it, I can't go any further.* I knew I was quitting before I'd reached my pain barrier. Gradually I realised that the time leading up to the two-hour mark was the hardest, when I would be in complete agony. Horrendous pain. It would feel as if my legs were crumbling beneath me. Then one day I got past it. *Fuck me*, I said to myself, almost in wonder. *I can go for ages.* It was like my body had reset itself. I came to look forward to stepping across that barrier, the moment when my body had become accustomed to the pain that was flooding through every limb and I got my second wind.

After a while I reached the point – whether it was in the gym, in combat carrying a stupid amount of weight or climbing Everest – when I could tell when the pain barrier was approaching. I realised that once you've understood what your body is capable of, how much it can endure, you find yourself welcoming discomfort. There's something amazing about knowing that no matter how much agony you're in *right now*, you're going to be back in the game before long.

You grit your teeth and get through it, and even the misery becomes a pleasure.

Anyone can do learn to do exactly the same thing as I did. Just like with your emotions, everybody's pain threshold will be different. It's your pain, own it. In order to under-stand your pain threshold you have to endure it for a period of time. So hit the gym and work out until your muscles ache, or go for a run that you know is longer and harder than you'd usually be comfortable with. To begin with you probably won't be able to make it through the pain barrier. You might not even get that close to it. That's fine; it's a work in progress.

Just as with everything else, you can't hope that at some point you'll magically be able to endure more pain than you did the previous day. The only way to do this that doesn't involve hooking yourself up to a morphine drip is to work hard. This means, inevitably, that you need to be prepared to commit to failure. But remember that no failure is absolute. Let's say you're trying to get used to swimming in the sea during winter. If you only manage to stay in the water for thirty seconds one day, you'll find you can last forty-five seconds the following day and a whole minute the day after. Incremental improvement is more solid and long-lasting than exponential leaps. You're slowly, patiently building foundations that will be very hard to shake.

KNOWLEDGE REALLY IS POWER

The more knowledge you acquire about pain and the way your body responds to it, the more power you'll have over it.

If you know that the pain isn't going to last forever – that at some point you *will* cross that pain threshold – then it becomes easier to endure. If you have a sense how much something is likely to hurt *before* you do it, then it becomes a less intimidating prospect: if you've coped with that pain before, then you know you're able to cope with it now.

The Australian version of *SAS: Who Dares Wins* features a backwards dive into a freezing cold lake. I know that the instant I hit the water I'm going to be in excruciating pain – so vicious it will make me gasp – for two to three minutes. But because I've done things like this before I know how long the pain will last, and how extreme it's likely to be. By contrast, the *idea* of it alone shits up a lot of the contestants. When you don't know how long you're going to be trapped inside that agonising feeling, it's so much more tempting to quit – or never even try at all.

It's always useful to remember that the battle against pain takes place in your brain as well as your body. People who've done Iron Mans will say that you can prepare for the physical challenge. It's the mental strain that is the hardest to cope with. If you've embarked on any kind of extremely demanding physical endeavour, the chances are that at some point you'll be energy depleted. This, clearly, has implications for your body, but it also presents a significant challenge to your mind. We shouldn't forget that our brain absorbs an enormous proportion of the calories we take in. When suddenly there's less of the sugar and glucose that we need, our brain struggles. We stop thinking rationally and start to fall apart. That's the moment you suddenly regret starting the race you're halfway through and begin to contemplate giving up.

If you know what the triggers are that might provoke this sort of thinking and have the tools in your pocket that allow you to reset, you might be able to find a way through. The advice I give in the chapters on building resilience and controlling your emotions is particularly relevant here (see Chapters 12 and 11).

Enlist all the allies you can in your struggle against the pain barrier. Although you're the only person who can actually cross that threshold, you don't have to do it completely alone. For instance, when you're tempted to give up, imagine that you've got people who love and support you sitting on your shoulder. What would they be saying to you to help you keep going?

Imagine how good you'll feel when you've completed the challenge and remind yourself what it means to you. When I was struggling through the rain in the Brecon Beacons, I kept on thinking about how amazing it would feel if I did pass Selection. That thought gave me the boost I needed at times when I was low and vulnerable. You can do the opposite too. I considered how angry and disappointed I'd be with myself if I gave up. I thought about how smug the faces of Bench and everyone else in 40 Commando who had doubted me would be when they learned that I'd chucked it in. It was something else that helped keep at bay the temptation to do something I knew I would later regret.

SHARE THE LOAD

The smarter you are with your approach to gruelling experiences, the more likely you are to succeed. Our body and brain are amazing resources. The trick is to learn how to deploy them as cleverly and effectively as possible.

When you're faced with an awesome physical and mental challenge, try to break it down into manageable chunks. Don't think about what you're doing next, don't waste energy. Be laser-focused on what's in front of you *right now*. One of the things that really helped me as I fought my way through the Brecon Beacons on Selection was that the whole ordeal was divided into different sections. My entire focus was on getting to the next checkpoint. It meant that my mind wasn't flooded with thoughts of the immensity of the task; it only had to consider manageable chunks of it.

The same is true of lots of the sorts of challenges you might be contemplating. A marathon is 26.2 miles, too much for our brains to contemplate. Break it down into small chunks. Challenge yourself to complete one mile at a time. It's not just that you'll have broken down an intimidating goal into much more easily achievable fragments; you'll also gain motivation from the constant stream of small but significant achievements. Psychologically, it's much more positive to consider all the things you've already done than it is to get too bogged down with contemplating what still lies ahead of you. Try to get as many wins under your belt as you can.

Once you've done that, work out which parts of the task are primarily mental and which are physical. Share that load. If it's a physical task, your brain can take a rest; if it's mental, then your body can have a break.

I might have two tasks in a day. One could be jumping backwards out of a helicopter. Lots of people would look at that as one intimidatingly large task and let themselves get overwhelmed by it. But I break it down. When you reduce it to its absolute essentials, all you have to do is commit to that one act. It's a confidence test that has nothing physical in it. It's all psychological. All it requires from me is ten seconds of mental effort and sufficient energy to walk over to the helicopter's door. You're not jumping, you're falling. It only becomes physical in any meaningful sense once you hit the water and have to start swimming to the other side. Then, once you're out of the water, it's psychological again. You've got to force yourself to stand there in the cold and get changed out of your soaking clothes as quickly as you can.

Yomping is physical when it's time to start running with the pack. As soon as the phase of walking uphill comes in, it starts being psychological – it's about putting one foot in front of the other. Once you reach the top and need to run down again, it's physical. Then at the checkpoint when I've got five to ten minutes to sort out my bearings it's a mental process once again. I switch off physically and switch on psychologically. At any given moment one part of me is able to rest, the other is laser-focused on the job in hand.

LESSONS

Everyone has a pain threshold. It's up to you to find yours.

Discover as much as you can about the way pain affects you. The more you know about how your body responds to extreme discomfort, the more control you'll be able to exert.

The war against pain is as much mental as it is physical. If you're ever contemplating taking on an awesome physical challenge, don't neglect your mental preparations.

You have a body and a mind – use them *both*. Share the load between your mental and physical faculties. If you can lean on your body to give your mind a rest, do it. You'll be grateful later.

CHAPTER 14

LEARN TO SAY NO

**Stand up for yourself, stand up to bullies
and discover the constructive power
of conflict.**

Caracas, Venezuela, 2012

The world is full of bad men doing bad things. Sometimes these villains are in combat gear or the black robes of an Islamist group. But what I learned after I'd left the military was a surprise to me: most of the time bad men are in suits.

The other thing I've learned is that oil sends some people mad. People will do anything for black gold; they'll lie, cheat, kill and try to fuck everybody else over. There are very few morals in those parts of that world where oil is king, and even fewer rules.

That's how I came to be sitting in an antiseptic boardroom in Caracas's business district. At face value it was just like any other business meeting: the gentle hiss of air-conditioning protecting us from the punishing heat outside, men with iron-grey hair in immaculately tailored Armani suits, expensive laptops, high-end refreshments.

But if you looked closer, you'd have been surprised by the line of three bruisers sitting against the far wall of the room. Their arms were crossed, their faces set in various types of scowls and their jackets visibly straining to contain the biceps within. They looked as if they'd be far more at home tearing phonebooks in half or chucking drunks out of nightclubs than delivering a PowerPoint presentation. The other thing out of place was, of course, me. I was sitting opposite them, beside a man named Javier whom I'd met a few weeks earlier.

Javier was a slight, elegant man who moved with an almost birdlike grace. I guessed he was in his early fifties, but he seemed younger. He was exquisitely, almost excessively polite, with the unruffled confidence of somebody who'd got through life without ever having to do anything he didn't want to. That, sadly for him, was about to change.

He was the CEO of a moderately sized oil company that had found itself on the wrong end of some bullying from a bigger one that wanted to take it over. Which, of course, is what businesses the world over do. Usually, however, there's a whole legal apparatus that governs the process and ensures a fair outcome. This was different. The big company didn't negotiate, they threatened. If they didn't get their way, they weren't going to walk away from the deal – they'd just destroy the smaller one. It wasn't much of a choice. All the smaller company could hope to do was keep a percentage of the enterprise they'd built. How big or small a percentage that was going to be would be determined in this series of meetings in Caracas. The fact that everybody was going to be in expensive suits gave a flimsy corporate sheen to what effectively was a mugging. I'd been brought in to escort Javier and the top brass to the meetings; I was back-up in case anything went badly awry during the discussions. I also had to make sure that they made it to the meetings at all.

Venezuela is one of the most oil-rich nations on the planet, but decades of corruption and incompetence have left it a shattered, lawless country. Crime is everywhere, everybody seems to have a price and the police are as rotten as everyone else. At the time there had been a rash of what were known as 'express kidnappings', where the criminals snatch somebody and then rather than hold out for a large ransom, simply demand the sort of figure – $50,000, say – that can be transferred in a matter of minutes. After that, everybody gets on with their business. The police at the very least turned a blind eye to it, and I'm sure a good few had their sticky mitts in numerous lucrative pies.

Violent gangs and powerful warlords controlled large swathes of the country, and Caracas crackled with menace. Every journey from our base outside the city, through the *barrios* that huddled on the precipitous hills around its perimeter and on to the glittering skyscrapers in the centre where our hotel was located, was fraught. We'd drive in against a soundtrack of running gun battles between heavily armed gangsters and government forces; we'd see burning cars belching acrid fumes, street crime, vicious muggings; and all the time we'd feel the hungry, desperate eyes watching us. Someone was always waiting for that one second when our guard slipped.

Everything had to be planned to the smallest detail. Our operating philosophy was that the shit probably would hit the fan, so it was in everybody's interests that we were suitably prepared. That's why they were paying four former elite operators to do the job. Most private security is basically just a question of making sure that weirdos – as well as passionate fans – can't get uncomfortably close to celebrities. This was all a bit different. We'd scope out small airstrips we could use to make a nifty exit, we'd arrange a network of safe houses we could go to in case we needed to lay low.

We always entered and exited our hotel via an underground doorway. I'd take the seat beside Javier. Another guy would be sitting behind the wheel of our car, ready to whisk us off at a moment's notice and a third would be somewhere close by, staring at his phone, ready for the call that would tell him to spring into action.

Our destination – the other company's headquarters – was a sparkling palace of glass and steel, a shocking contrast to the shambolic decay that characterised so much of the city. Everything here was new and blisteringly hi-tech, the sort of place designed both to impress and intimidate. It was also safer and more impenetrable than Fort Knox. There were key systems, doors that locked with a frighteningly efficient hiss, and, wherever you turned, black-clad security guards. As we entered I felt frustrated all over again at the fact that the local laws meant that we weren't allowed weapons. If things got really bad there was a Venezuelan in our team who was licensed to carry – we saw him as our travelling armoury. Except, of course, he was now on the other side of this battery of security measures. No matter how keen he was to come to our rescue, there wasn't much he could do beyond creating a diversion that would hopefully last long enough to enable us to get our client to safety.

I'd clocked all this as I walked behind Javier, who floated happily along. I could have sworn he was actually whistling to himself. My eyes flitted around constantly, looking to see which elevator we could take if we needed to make a run for it or what doors we could use. Normally in these situations you could see a route out. This time I knew that that we'd be searching for a weak point for a million years and still never find it. I texted the lads. If things went tits up in the next few minutes, I told them, we were stuck.

We were ushered into the meeting room, where we sank into our seats. Almost before we'd got our bearings, the guys from the other company had got things moving. Their leader was an imposing man with slicked-back jet-black hair reminding me, absurdly, of an otter. He was sleek and slippery, and could neither stand still nor stop talking. In somebody else, this might have come across as nerves, but he didn't appear unsettled in any way. It was more that he seemed determined to dominate the room and everybody in it as completely as possible. He was as friendly and subtle as a Gatling gun, and only a tiny bit quieter.

My Spanish is limited to what you need to order a beer, so I couldn't understand the detail of what he said. But that didn't really matter, because there was no mistaking the tone. His voice was harsh, guttural and accompanied by incessant gestures. Every so often he would lean close to Javier, so close that my employer must have been able to tell exactly what the Otter had eaten for breakfast. It was clear he was trying to provoke Javier, and yet Javier remained impassive, which only seemed to enrage the other man. Voices rose. Fingers were pointed. That initial tension was replaced by something that felt like naked aggression.

In theory I was just a PA, which probably would have been a stretch at the best of times, but it seemed even more ridiculous because I was as heavily muscled as anybody else in that room, had a full beard and you could see tattoos creeping beneath the cuffs of my shirt. The other side made it clear that as far as they were concerned my presence was a bit of a farce, but they didn't actually say anything. What could they say?

I was painfully aware of the security lined up against the opposite wall. If something kicked off it would be them, not their beautifully dressed bosses, who'd be up there causing us trouble. Every so often I'd give them a brief stare, meet their gaze, just to show them that I was present and fully aware of the situation. It wasn't pointless machismo, it wasn't dick-swinging. It was to say, 'I know why I'm here, you know why you're here. I'm here to look after my client, you're here to look after yours. This isn't personal, it's professional.' It was an affirmation of mutual respect.

I was hyper-conscious of the energy in the room, both mine and theirs. I could see that we were all doing as much as we could to show that we weren't alarmed by the vicious turn the meeting had taken. I knew that I had to hold my nerve. Without doing anything overt, I needed to show that I wasn't intimidated and I wasn't going to back down.

Just as the meeting seemed about to explode into a massacre, it came to an end. Javier stood up, made an almost imperceptible nod of his head to me, and we left. The second we stepped out of the building's front door I noticed I was soaked in sweat, my heart was racing and every part of my body seemed to be firing with adrenaline. Everyone else in our party looked almost traumatised by the tension and anger of the last few minutes, except one. Javier was gently dabbing at his temples with a handkerchief, but otherwise seemed untroubled. What the fuck was he on? 'Well,' he said, in his lightly accented but otherwise flawless English, 'that was an interesting start.'

The process was repeated again and again over the next six weeks. Each time it got worse. Tempers got more frayed, the levels of aggression rose and rose. And yet Javier rose serenely above it all. There were moments when I couldn't believe what I was seeing. Still, even if he wasn't worried, we very definitely were. Ahead of the final meeting we decided to activate the safehouses and air strips: it had begun to seem inevitable that we'd need to use them. In the evenings we'd be studying maps of the city, trying to make sure that if we needed to get out of it fast, we could.

The final meeting began like all the others. We'd been escorted up to the boardroom by the silent, black-clad security guards. There was no small talk, nobody offered us drinks; we just got straight down to the matter at hand.

I took my seat at the table and sat quietly as the bosses began to talk. Occasionally I'd scribble something meaningful in the notepad I'd brought with me. It probably looked fairly official from across the table, but all anybody who actually leafed through its pages would have found were some scribbled smiley faces.

By this point the Otter and his men had prepared a contract. I never actually had it in my hands, but from the animated arguments that erupted after Javier and his team had read the document, its terms were obviously very much in the bigger company's favour. What was also clear was that they weren't in much of a mood to negotiate the terms. Although I don't think they ever actually said as much, their message had been sharpened to a nasty point: sign the contract or we'll shoot you all.

Even this wasn't enough to persuade our boys. They refused point blank. Javier remained polite but steely, and his other guys went along with him. By that point I was just willing them to sign the fucking thing. My phone was now in my hand, my thumb hovering over the button that would send a message to the men I had waiting outside the building: Code Red.

The room suddenly soured with tension. I had the ludicrous thought that perhaps, having survived so many hardcore missions with the SBS, I was going meet my maker here, in a Venezuelan boardroom, among cafetieres, porcelain cups and Danish pastries. Javier gestured to the contract, then indicated he'd be taking it away to read. I stood up, Javier stared at me for a second. I nodded at him, then he picked the pile of paper up. There was a scrape of chairs on the immaculately polished parquet and the other side got to their feet, almost in unison. Behind the Otter, his security bristled with the strain that still gripped the whole room.

The two CEOs stared at each other like they wanted to smash the other man's face in. It was the first time I'd ever seen Javier look anything other than serene, which alone was enough to scramble my mind. Normally, even in the hairiest moments in Afghanistan and beyond, I'd a clear sense of what might happen. The odds might be stacked against us, but at least I'd know what we needed to do. But right now I had no idea which way the situation would go, and no clue as to how we could escape.

There was another incomprehensible volley of Spanish, followed by Javier replying sharply with a word that I did understand: 'No.' Everything immediately fell frighteningly silent. Javier's defiance seemed to echo around the room. It seemed as if the air had suddenly got thinner, and I became painfully conscious of a bead of sweat dribbling slowly down my forehead. Fuck. Fuck. Fuck. What *was* he thinking? This did not look good. Doing everything I could to keep my face seeming as calm and unruffled as possible, I scanned the room for a weapon. The only thing that looked even vaguely promising was a fountain pen that someone had placed on the table. I found myself wondering how sharp it was.

And then the two men exchanged a simple nod. Javier turned on his heels and made as if to leave the room, although where he thought he was heading I have no fucking idea. I followed him – because what else could I do? I was as useful as a lump of butter. If something went off, there was no point in me being there. We got as far as the first security door, which was as impassable now as it had been thirty minutes earlier. At that point a little dude who'd sat in silence during the whole meeting scampered out, waved his key card over the sensor and the doors hissed open.

AN HOUR LATER we were sitting safely in the plush seats of Javier's air-conditioned limousine.

I was desperate to find out what had happened. Finally, I blurted out a question: 'Why did you say No? Why didn't you just give in?'

Javier smiled. He was immaculate, his shirt uncreased, not a hair out of place. There was no sign of the immense pressure he'd been under only minutes before. 'He was a bully, Anthony,' he said. 'If I had not said No, he would have sensed that I was weak, and he would have taken and taken and taken until there was nothing left.'

'Weren't you afraid?' I asked him.

'Yes, of course,' he said, smiling again, a bit more shyly this time. 'But I could not have lived with myself if I had not tried.'

A LOT ABOUT the situation left a bitter taste in my mouth. Javier was a very rich man when I first met him and he was still a very rich man by the time I left the country. But it was hard to see what had happened as a victory. Walking out of the office without signing the contract had got him a better deal than if he'd given in immediately, but the bare bones of it was that he'd had his company stolen from him.

The whole sequence of events felt like the opposite of everything I'd been used to during my years in the armed forces. Nothing of note had actually happened. Nobody had pulled a gun or even come to blows. We'd been to several meetings, there had been some arguments, we'd walked away at the end. And yet as I sank into my seat on the plane that took us home I realised how psychologically and physically drained I was. It was as if I'd been on a three-day tier one operation.

At the same time, I was inspired by the way Javier had stood up for himself in such a daunting situation. He had showed me the power of saying No.

THERE'S AN AMAZING power in saying No. It's a way of resisting other people's expectations, of saying, 'Enough is enough.' And yet so many of us appear to be unaware of its potency. We run ourselves ragged trying to accommodate other people's unreasonable demands. We say, 'Don't worry, I can try this' or 'Leave it with me, I'll sort it' when we know that the real answer is 'No, I don't want to do that' or 'No, I'm not putting up with that,' but we're too anxious about hurting another person's feelings or disappointing them. And some of us are so afraid of conflict that we'll never say a word to the boss who's bullying us or the parent who makes us feel as if nothing we do is ever good enough. Instead we lead miserable, crushed existences. Often we're so unhappy that we pass our suffering on to the people that we claim to care for most.

It doesn't need to be like this. Once you've overcome the fear of the consequences of saying No, once you've learned how to stand up for yourself, you'll be liberated. Of course it's fucking scary and hard. If it wasn't, you wouldn't have avoided it for so long. It will probably involve upset, it will definitely involve hard work, but the long-term consequences of putting up with things will far outweigh the short-term discomfort of confrontation.

HOW MUCH ARE YOU WILLING TO TAKE?

Let's say you're the sort of person who hates confrontation. You avoid it all costs. Maybe it's because the mere *idea* of conflict seems too intimidating. Or perhaps you're just afraid that talking honestly will end up hurting somebody's feelings. Whenever a situation arises that you know might involve a showdown, you find a way of dodging it. You rely on those ancient excuses: 'It's not the perfect moment' or 'It's not the right time'. Instead you let things carry on as they are. Your friend keeps on talking down to you, or your colleague keeps taking credit for the work you do, and you just suck it all up, no matter how unhappy it makes you. After all, it's the easier thing to do, isn't it?

I can understand that perspective. But I also think it's crucial that you leave it behind. This is your only life. You don't get to live it again. If you've got a problem with someone and it's affecting your happiness and well-being, why don't you tell them? If their behaviour is damaging you psychologically, why wouldn't you do something about it? Why put up with that misery? Is that how you want to spend the rest of your time on the planet? Do you want to look back and say, 'If only I'd said something earlier, everything would have been so much better'?

And are you happy about the knock-on effect that your unhappiness has on those who love and cherish you? Are you OK with the fact that one person is making not only you but your wife and kids miserable because you haven't got the courage to confront them?

As much as you might want it to, the problem isn't going to disappear by itself. Ultimately, it's only you who holds the answer. Only you can do anything about the situation. It's up to you to tell yourself, *I'm suffering, other people around me are suffering. I have to do something.*

So come up with a game plan. Tell yourself, on Monday morning I'm going to knock on my boss's door and let him know how I feel. And remember this: everything you think you know about conflict is wrong.

ON *SAS: Who Dares Wins* you see me shouting at every-body in sight, but that's just the persona I adopt for the programme. It's not me. It's just what I have to do to push the recruits to where they need to be, and to make good TV.

In my day-to-day life I'm far softer. Particularly when it comes to those hard conversations where you need to do the sort of straight talking that you know could end up hurting the other person, I'll always be respectful. I don't shout and scream. I'm far more interested in being empathetic and sensitive. What I aim to do is find a collaborative approach that emphasises the things we have in common, our shared goals.

The word 'confrontation' carries a lot of meaning for us. It implies an aggressive exchange of opinions, it suggests that things could get personal, even nasty. But this doesn't have to be the case. It's just a word that describes a situation in which two people have two different sets of values, or two different ways of seeing the world. There isn't anything inherently violent about it.

I find this to be a useful way of stripping the idea of conflict of the terror it holds for many people. These aren't situations to be rushed. When I find myself faced by someone who's behaving in a way that makes me uncomfortable or unhappy, I always begin by giving the other person enough time to get to that point where *they* want to change. Sometimes they'll recognise the problem and try to do something about it. If that doesn't happen, if they keep ignoring the situation, then it's time for some brutal honesty.

Look at the problem deeply. Think about how it's affecting you, but also the impact it's having on them. It's far better to frame your intervention as an act of sympathy – somebody trying to help – rather than it coming across as an attack. Focus on the positives that will emerge from that person changing. Offer them a positive reason to change. Show them how their behaviour is impacting not only you and others in their life, but also themselves. The really important thing to bear in mind when you're talking to those that you love – like parents, siblings or partners – is to be kind. Show them that what you're doing is out of love: 'I'm saying this *because* I care.'

Two of my kids are into their teens now and that teenage attitude is already starting to come in. A point came when I had to be honest with them. 'You're becoming horrible,' I told them. 'Do you know where that's going to get you? Soon people aren't going to want to be around you. I'm your dad. I love you with all my heart, I don't want to see a hair on your head hurt, and yet even *I* don't want to be around you at the moment. This isn't you. I haven't brought you up to be like this. Just think about it.'

Rage rarely achieves anything. I'm not naïve. I know that some situations will escalate into an argument. But why choose to *begin* an encounter that way? Why embroil yourself in an unnecessary fracas? So try not to be angry. Take the emotion away. Just present the situation as calmly and fairly as you can. 'This is a problem and it's really affecting me.' Be aware not just of what you say, but *how* you say it. Maintain eye contact. Make sure your voice is firm and serious; this isn't small talk.

If your kid is being bullied by another child at school, call the other kids' parents and tell them what's happening in a calm, measured way. Don't start screaming accusations down the phone the second they answer. You're not going to war against each other, you're trying to fix a shared problem. Javier was a master at this approach. Everything he said to the Otter was calm and thought through. I don't think he raised his voice once. And yet when it came to saying No, he was uncompromising. The other side were left in no doubt that he was utterly serious.

I DON'T WANT to give the false impression that these sorts of conversations are easy. No matter how careful you are to find the perfect form of words or the perfect way of expressing yourself, you can't control how the other person will react.

So don't be surprised if to begin with they're defensive or aggressive. Honesty is hard – for everybody involved. And that's especially true when it's between two human beings who love each other. People don't like to hear the truth. But it's when you get that friction that you *know* you've hit a nerve. If somebody reacts really badly when you tell them that their behaviour is out of order, it shows that deep down they're already aware of the situation.

They'll probably go away and think about what you've said, and gradually they'll understand. It's always going to be a slow process. When you ask somebody to adjust their view of the world and their place in it, they're inevitably going to resist. Who wants to be told that they've been hurting others? Who likes to have boundaries reset? Give them time, give them space. Let them break it down and really absorb this fresh information. If they're honest with themselves, they'll find the answer.

What's also important to bear in mind is that even if the encounter doesn't quite work out like you think it will, the fact of getting something off your chest is already a win. The confrontation might have made you feel uncomfortable, upset or guilty, but you'll have learned something. You'll have gone somewhere you haven't dared travel before. You'll be changed by the experience – and as soon as you've managed this once, you'll find that saying No gets easier and easier. And you'll also see that it will change the way others see you.

If you can't ever find a way of saying No, other people will take advantage of you. They'll see you as soft and weak, and they won't respect you. They know that they can do what they want to you and always get away with it.

But if you're willing to stand up for yourself, if you can make it clear where your boundaries are and that you won't tolerate them being broken, people will respect you more. Javier's willingness to say No sent an unmistakeable message to the bigger company: you cannot trample on me. It worked. Confrontation is another route to growth.

GET OUT OF YOUR HEAD

Very often, the person who is making you miserable in your personal or professional life will have no idea at all that they're affecting you.

We all think and feel differently. There's stuff that would drive me absolutely crazy that you might be able to brush off like it's nothing. But if it doesn't bother you, how the hell are you going to know what sort of effect it has on me unless I tell you? Perhaps your boss is unaware of how their abrasive management style comes across, or your mother doesn't realise her constant stream of parenting advice leaves you feeling undermined. Take this into account when you speak to them.

Say, for example, your boss chewed you out in front of your colleagues in a meeting the previous week. When you walk into their office, show them that you understand where they're coming from: 'In that last meeting you raised your voice and spoke to me in a pretty condescending way. I don't think it was needed in that particular situation. If you had a problem, maybe you could have just pulled me to one side after the meeting was over? We could have spoken about it face to face rather than you making me feel that way in public. I know you're the boss and you have your own way of communicating with your team, but this felt like it had crossed into something personal. It made me feel really uncomfortable.'

The chances are that they'll have been completely oblivious to the situation – most of us are wrapped up in our own lives, we don't really understand how we come across or the effect we have on others. They'll say: 'That's just me, that's who I am, that's how I deal with things. But if that's how you feel, if me talking to you differently will help you work better, then I'm pleased you came to me. I'm sorry, I didn't want to make you uncomfortable.'

I've found that employing empathy is also useful if you find yourself in an argument with somebody. Attempt to understand what is pushing them into the confrontation. What matters to them so much that they're willing to lock horns with you? Show them that you understand their perspective. Ask yourself: what must they be going through to behave like that? What is their life like? If you at least try to empathise with them, then you might be able to find some common ground. If you can locate that meeting place which helps you see each other as human beings with shared interests and concerns, then a lot of anger and rage falls away very quickly. Instead of being opponents butting heads, you're collaborators trying to solve a problem together.

YOUR NEGATIVITY ISN'T MY PROBLEM

I despise bullies. I hate seeing people being bullied or taken advantage of. I hate seeing human beings manipulating other human beings.

My hatred for that sort of character has got me into trouble more than once. If I see someone bullying another person, I just can't sit back and let it go. Back in the day, I think the majority of people would be like me: they'd say something or intervene in some other way. Now they're petrified to do so because they know that sticking up for another human being could have all sorts of complicated consequences. Our society has encouraged that reluctance: the message we get is, 'It's none of your business.'

So my more practical advice for dealing with bullies would always be: if you can, steer well clear of them. It's very rare that anything positive will come from an encounter with a bully. I'll always tell my kids to ignore them. But there are things you can do if avoiding them isn't possible because you share an office with them,

When you boil it down, bullies want to play mind games with you. The majority of bullying is psychological. So it's essential that you don't overthink your encounters with bullies. Why waste hours of your valuable time contemplating somebody who's riddled with negativity? What can it possibly achieve other than making you miserable and stressed? I guarantee you this: they'll not be spending a single second thinking about you. They're not going to be sitting there saying: 'Oh, I wonder how I can make *his* life a misery.' But you'll make their day if you let on that you've spent the night beforehand agonising about them. It tells them they've got a hold over you.

Ultimately, they're opportunists. They're not criminal masterminds plotting an audacious raid on a bank; they're just bums who take advantage of open windows. If they can get away with something, they will. Bullies act up because they want attention, or are struggling with insecurities or other issues that lead to them pushing their negativity outwards onto other people. Your response is their fuel. It's almost never personal. They just want you to help them exorcise their demons. The best thing you can do is to not offer them the opportunities they're always on the lookout for.

But if you do find yourself on the wrong end of that sort of behaviour, begin by remembering that it's the other person's problem. Relinquish any responsibility for the negativity they're trying to thrust into your hands: 'Your negativity isn't my problem, mate.'

Don't rise to their bait. Instead, do what you can to gain control of the situation.

Bullies like to feel as if they're getting their own way. In Venezuela we worked hard to give the other side the illusion of a complete surrender without actually having to give any more away than we could stomach. We fed them ideas, then persuaded them that they'd come up with them in the first place. The more you can manipulate them without them realising that they're being manipulated, the better.

And what often works for me is killing the other person with kindness. Negative people *want* you to get worked up and upset because that's what they feed off. That's the fuel they need to carrying on firing their negativity. So when I get shit from people for 'selling my soul', I try to disarm them by admitting straight away that they're right, I *am* selling my soul. Then I tell them why: 'Everything I do is so I can put a roof over my family's head. I'd give away anything, do *anything* for my family. Wouldn't you?'

I start off by agreeing with them, and we end up in a completely different place to where we'd started. Suddenly we're relating to each other. These sorts of situations are why I'll never stop going on about how important it is to be sociable: make sure you have good manners; be kind in your interactions; be the sort of person who can get on with other people. It's paid off for me time and time again.

Of course, unfortunately some people are cunts who don't deserve anything except a good hiding. You can't do anything for them. They certainly can't do anything for you. So the only thing you can do is to do yourself a favour and stay the fuck away.

BE SMARTER THAN THE SITUATION

I wasn't in Venezuela to stir anything up. My job was to keep everything as calm as possible. That's what my client wanted, and I had to ensure that our energies were synced. If he was completely irate and I was slumped on my chair chilling out, it would look as if something was wrong.

So my behaviour was crucial. If I'd been edgier or less in control, the security on the other side of the room would have noticed. If I'd panicked, I'd have landed Javier in a pile of shit.

I use the same approach in any situation that threatens to get out of hand. First, read the room. Start thinking and assessing as soon as you can. Look out for posture, body-language. What are they trying to communicate? Are they trying to assert themselves?

Do what you can to calm things down. Remember that nothing good will come from you throwing more fuel onto the fire. I learned that the hard way. For too long I believed that the best response to provocation was more aggression. And I carried on believing this until my attitude got me sent to prison.

Now I always try to remind myself that I'm smart enough to avoid violent confrontation, which is always going to be the worst-case scenario. When both parties have lost their shit, that's it: there's no way back. If you have to, don't be afraid to turn around and walk away. Nobody has ever made a good decision after the red mist has descended.

If you have a bit of an altercation while driving, try to take the heat out of the situation. If you know that you're in the wrong, admit it, even if their reaction is disproportionate to what's happened. What do you really have to lose? 'I apologise, I'm not from round here, I wanted to go straight on but found myself in the wrong lane. I didn't mean to cut you up.' If you can control your own emotions, you'll be able to control the situation.

LESSONS

If you never stand up for yourself, nobody will respect you. Is that how you want to live?

Confrontation doesn't need to be aggressive. Take the emotion out of the situation. You don't need to attack the other person; just let them know that you have a problem and you want them to help you solve it.

You're responsible for what you say and how you say it. You're not responsible for how the other person reacts. Be as kind and considerate as possible, but don't let the fear of hurting their feelings stop you from telling them what they need to hear. If they get upset, that's up to them.

A bully's negativity isn't your problem. All that bullies want is to pass their negativity on to other people. Just ignore them. Don't give them the chance to infect you with their misery.

Don't be a bomb-thrower. There's almost no scenario in civilian life to which violence is the answer. Always do what you can to de-escalate the situation. Don't be too proud to apologise. Don't be afraid to walk away.

CHAPTER 15

LOOK AFTER YOUR BEARD

You're an individual, one of a kind;
celebrate what makes you special.

ONE OF THE reasons I wanted to go on Selection was because I knew that, if I passed, I'd be able to grow my hair and beard. I liked the non-conformist reputation of the Special Forces, the way that going against the grain was encouraged. They weren't hung up on whether you shaved or not, or if you had hair creeping out the bottom of your helmet.

The Marines insisted on short back and sides. They were very regimented – and that's why they're such a brilliant unit. But I was beginning to find that relentless discipline stifling. There were too many rules and regulations, too much control over where you went, what you did and how you did it. I wanted to be able to step out of the crowd and create my own identity, not just share it with everyone else who wore the same beret as me. I wanted to carry on growing – if I'd stayed in the Marines there would have been parts of myself that I'd never be able to unlock.

As soon as I passed, that was it. I could do whatever I wanted with my hair, my body, my clothes and – of course – my beard. As far as I was concerned, as long as I did my job on the battlefield it didn't matter if I was scruffy or wearing mismatched gear. I didn't care about being a perfect camp soldier. That's not what I'd joined up to do. I had extremely high expectations of my performance on the battlefield. What I did, or how I dressed once I was back at the base, was irrelevant.

I loved the fact that you could wear anything, and I wanted to make sure I stood out. I'd turn up in operational gear mixed with desert stuff, like sand-coloured boots, or American uniforms. You could take the piss, get tattoos up your neck (I reckon I probably had more ink than anybody else in the Special Forces at the time). And I liked the way that when you walked past regular soldiers in their green camo and black boots you'd see them clock you. They'd rarely say anything, but you could tell they were thinking, *Who the fuck is* he?

The beard has become a huge part of my identity and I'm not sure I'd ever consider shaving it off. I have actually been offered money, a *lot* of money, to do that. Even though it was for charity I realised I just couldn't do it. But some nights I have dreams – which stop just short of being nightmares – that my beard has been shaved off. I wake with a start, convinced that I'm going to have to hide away for two weeks growing it back. Luckily it grows pretty quickly and I don't need to worry about patches here or there. Oddly enough, I've got the army to thank for that. They don't care if you can barely grow bumfluff, they insist that you shave until your cheeks shine. Which meant that from the age of sixteen I was scraping away at my face with a razor every day – a pretty nasty experience at the time, but one which has ended up making a significant difference to me now. It's strange how life works out.

IF YOU'RE READING this chapter hoping for my inside tips on beard maintenance, then I'm afraid I'm going to disappoint you. I don't have any special tricks or routines. I don't oil my beard or anything like that, I just keep it nicely combed and wash it the same way I do the rest of my hair. My only thing is that I won't let anybody else cut it, not even Emilie. (That might be because she prefers me without it – according to her, it makes me look ten years younger. She likes a five o'clock shadow, and not much more.)

But I can tell you what having a beard means to me. I've found that my beard is a good way of opening myself up to the world, like a sign telling others what sort of headspace I'm in. Some people hide behind their beards. I'm the opposite. It's liberating. When I was on tour it would grow out into a big bushy affair, and the same happens in the gap between filming shows for TV. If my hair and beard are cropped short – when I shave my cheeks and grow a kind of Leonidas beard – it's my way of signalling that I'm feeling sharp and mean business. If both hair and beard are wild and long, it's a sign that I'm feeling carefree.

I first grew the beard when I was only twenty-six, an age when you're still figuring out who you really are and what you want from life. If I look back at who I was then, the beard was a kind of waymarker. It was me saying, *I'm on my way to becoming a different kind of person.* Even now, I'm trying to add layers to my identity. I want to celebrate my individuality – and silly as it might sound, my beard is absolutely central to that. For the last two decades it's been an expression of who I am and how I feel. It's been a symbol of my desire to stand out from the crowd and do things differently. You might not like it, but it's part of me and I'm fucking proud of it.

And that's the last of this book's fifteen rules. We're all unique in our own beautiful, messy, imperfect, amazing ways. That's something I think we should celebrate. Your individuality is something to be cherished and fought for. Don't be afraid to be different. Don't apologise for who you are, or the clothes you wear, the food you eat, the books you read, the body you have or the values you hold. Grow a beard, wear a dress, join the circus, form a band. Do whatever the fuck you want. If those things are authentic to you, if they're a true reflection of how you think and feel, then you should never, ever be ashamed of them. Be proud. Be you.

ACKNOWLEDGEMENTS

THANKS TO JACK Fogg and Jordan Johnson for making magic happen yet again, and to Josh Ireland for helping me get my thoughts onto the page. I'm really grateful to everyone at YMU, and also to Max and Gaby at Dundas. I couldn't do what I do without you guys.

My wife Emilie is the most amazing partner any man could wish for. I love that we're still going on this journey through life together. I also cannot forget my brothers Jez, Arf, Paddy and Mike Morris. And my uncle Andy. The truest family I know.

A good life is a life full of good friends. I'm lucky to be able to call Carl Froch, Tony Bellew, Wayne Bridge, Liam Payne, Rebel Wilson and Locksmith my mates. Thank you all for being there during the stormy weather. We shall enjoy the sun together soon enough!

And, Nims Dai, you're one of a kind.

Thank you all. You mean more to me than you could ever guess.